JAMES R. GREGG, O.D.

the
sportsman's
eye

How to Make Better Use of
Your Eyes in the Outdoors

WINCHESTER PRESS

Library of Congress Catalog Card Number 73-150385

ISBN 0-87691-035-5

Published by Winchester Press
460 Park Avenue, New York 10022

Printed in the United States of America

Design by Diana Hrisinko

acknowledgments

Some of the material in this book appeared in various outdoor magazines. Credit is especially given to Field and Stream, Guns and Ammo, Plane and Pilot, Skin Diver and Better Camping. Photos came willingly from many sources, from individuals, institutions, and manufacturers; these sources are credited with the appropriate reproductions. Special thanks go to the Los Angeles College of Optometry, the Vision Conservation Institute of California, and the American Optometric Association for supplying assistance and materials.

preface

As a boy in high school, I envisaged a career in the outdoors. Life for me didn't turn out that way, not quite at least, until writing this book, in a vicarious sort of a way, almost made that dream come true.

It has been my extreme good fortune to have spent a great deal of time outdoors, even though my work as an optometrist and teacher is about as confined to the indoors as any can be. Yet it gave me freedom to maneuver long and frequent vacations. These became a sort of second "vocation" as I began writing about them.

There were no objections from my family. My wife, Bernice, who loves nothing more than a crackling campfire on a soft summer evening, was constantly ready to go. Ron, who can catch fish where there aren't any, and Janell, who always wanted to see what was at the end of a trail, were enthusiastic for any trip I could dream up.

That family of mine really gets credit for a book like this. They let me pull them around from Alaska to Key West and from Hawaii to Nova Scotia. We tried every sport in the book—mountain climbing, skiing, golf, canoeing, archery, boating—everything but flying our own plane, though we used plenty of other people's.

This book then embodies a great sense of personal achievement for me. It offers a lot of information about vision which I believe many people should know. If they do know more about their eyes and how to use them, they will enjoy the outdoors even more. Then I have done some good.

There is an ulterior motive too. People who love the outdoors, respect and protect it. The more of them there are who feel that way, the longer and better can nature exist in her fragile state. I hope it stays that way because there is so much more yet to do and to see.

January 25, 1971 JAMES R. GREGG

contents

the sportsman's eye

part one

about
your
vision

chapter **1**

introduction

Over the centuries, man has learned to use his eyes effectively in a great variety of outdoor environments and to make sense out of a bewildering array of visual images. How well he can do this depends upon the nature of his visual mechanism and also on his ability to correct any errors of sight that hamper his vision. He has by now become very skillful at adapting vision to outdoor seeing needs, and this is fortunate since at least half of the population requires some kind of visual aid for use outdoors.

Besides correcting defective sight, man has developed certain perceptual skills that quite possibly give him greater seeing prowess in nature than his ancestors ever possessed. On the other hand, his civilized, citified, and regulated life has restricted his background of experience about things in the outdoors. Most men need to sharpen their seeing skills in order to perform better outdoors. Fortunately, they can work at this with potentially good results.

The Visual Environment

The environment in which modern man operates creates some problems. He flies 30,000 feet above the earth and swims far below the surface of the sea. He plays golf in the California desert, skis the Rockies in deep snow, hikes in the rain forests of Alaska's panhandle, swims at Florida's white sand beaches. And many men do most or all of these things.

Rain, wind, sleet, snow and fog change the seeing environment in a few minutes time. Not only does brightness drop, so does visibility. A whole new set of perceptual reference factors has to be called into play as the light fails at evening time. In darkness, visual clues take on a different significance.

Man learns to interpret the meaning of the outside world by blobs of light entering his eye. Radiant light energy can only vary in three ways: intensity—which produces brightness; wavelength—which produces color; and the angle at which the light enters the eye—which tells something about location. From these clues alone, he must get meaning.

The range of brightness, for example, is so great in the outdoors and the maximum intensity so high that the eye does a lot better if it has some protection from glare. The difference in brightness from deepest shade to brilliant sunlight is as much as 10,000 times. Even though the eye has remarkable ability to automatically adjust to the amount of light, one of the big obstacles to seeing clearly outdoors is glare.

Long ago man invented devices to protect his eyes from overbrightness of the sun. Various materials such as wood, bone, skin, and metal were used by cutting narrow slits or punching holes in a piece shaped to fit in front of the eyes. Tinted lenses made of colored quartz have also long been used, dating back many centuries before the invention of spectacles about 1300 A.D. But until recently man could rest his eyes at night, for artificial lighting was not sufficiently developed to affect his habits greatly.

Now all has changed and man travels day and night and in visual environments as simple as pitch blackness in the woods and as diverse as the myriad of lights on a city freeway. By extending the day into the night, he greatly enlarged his seeing environment. And in daylight endless pavement, close-cropped lawns, gleaming walls, broad

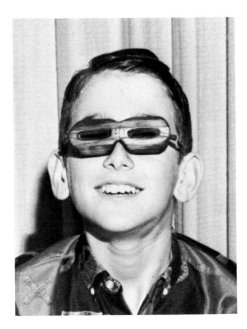

Eskimo goggles made of wood with leather straps to hold them in place. Slits are charred to reduce reflection and give maximum glare protection.

open fields, shrinking groundcover and fewer trees have increased glare tremendously. In addition, man moves in a world of boats, cars, and airplanes whose shiny surfaces reflect light into his eyes.

Some of this visual environment is potentially harmful to man. Infrared rays, the long wavelengths just beyond red in the visible spectrum, and ultraviolet, the short ones just below blue, can damage the tissues of the eye. The optical surfaces of the eye, the cornea and the crystalline lens, serve as filters to block out some of the invisible rays. So do properly compounded tinted lenses. It is generally agreed that some protection from excessive ultraviolet may be desirable. There is less agreement about infrared. But in some degree, man must be careful about exposure to the visual environment; there are limits to his tolerance. For example, long exposure to the winter sun can produce snow blindness.

The eye also has to make sense out of all of the color differences that it sees. Everything in nature is colorless. The eye sees color because objects reflect only certain wavelengths. Color is a psychological phenomena. If only the short end of the visible spectrum is

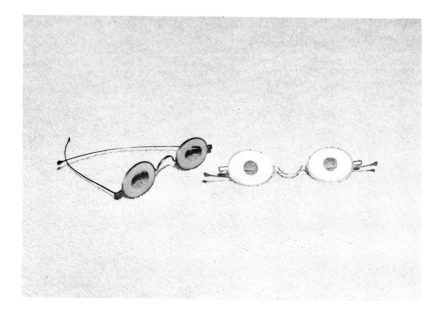

Hunting glasses of the early 1900's. The central openings are tinted glass; the periphery is designed to block the sunlight.

reflected, the objects look to be some kind of blue, the long wavelengths look red, and the middle ones green or yellow. By various combinations of wavelengths, it is possible to produce some 500,000 different shades and hues.

Brightness, size, and background all complicate seeing color. Nature has taken advantage of this by coloring animals so they resemble their background. The sharp-eyed outdoorsman learns to recognize this. And it is quite likely that how well he can do so is at least in some degree dependent upon the kind of visual references he has developed.

Visual References

There have been some fascinating studies dealing with the susceptibility of people with different cultural backgrounds to certain optical illusions. One of these studies used a test object of two lines equal in length with one placed vertically and the other horizontally

—the so-called vertical-horizontal illusion. Plains people, those who lived nomadic existence on the plains, always judged the vertical line longer. City dwellers made the same error but not so markedly. However, people who spent their lives in tall forests, as the pygmies in Africa, were not affected by the vertical illusion.

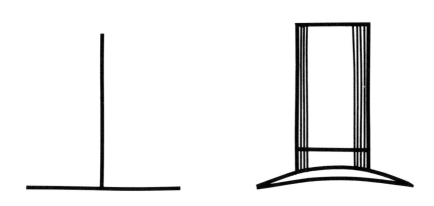

The vertical-horizontal illusion. Is the vertical height of these two figures greater than their horizontal width? Get out a ruler and check.

Few scientists would wish to make flat predictions based on these studies, but they would admit the suggestion that cultural background might influence how a person sees. It may well be then that man sees in terms of what he is accustomed to. The man who spends 90 percent of his waking hours within the four walls of his office and his home is going to have some problems perceiving across an endless prairie. Except when he is driving a car, and must judge relatively limited distances, he rarely looks at great expanses of space.

The patterns in nature are helter-skelter compared to those man creates. Curtains hang in straight lines, wallpaper usually has rows of figures, and the pages of a book have right angle corners. There is no such man made regularity in a tree, a river, or a mountain. The spots on the leopard, the plumage of a quail, the structure of a leaf have pattern but hardly computer-like symmetry; indeed, no two are alike.

The outdoor environment has been made from a different set of blueprints than those man used to create his artificial world, and this raises an interesting question. As man spends more of his time in buildings and in an architecturally created world, will this alter his ability to perceive in the natural environment? If it does, he will have to work even harder at sharpening his outdoor perceptual skills.

The Eye of the Outdoorsman

Why can the guide spot game long before his hunter client? Does he have superior eyesight? Or can he simply make better use of vision because of his vast background of experience in the outdoors and his intimate knowledge of animal life?

Visual scientists have racked their brains over these questions for years—this is the age-old controversy over the influence of heredity versus learning on human performance. The factor of natural selection undoubtedly has an influence in choosing an outdoor career. The guide who cannot tell the difference between a buffalo and a barn door will not get many calls for his services. Only those people who have good eyesight, or can get it, generally go into a business which places a premium on seeing ability.

Though the matter has never been studied statistically, it is possible that most outdoorsmen, both amateur and professional, have good natural eyesight. They may have a certain kind of ability to see at great distances in a vast array of environments that is superior to the average person, for they must judge distance, light and color, perceive a mass of forms with remarkable precision. This is far different from the kind of vision it takes to perform close work at desk, bench, lathe, or in school. Rarely do professionals in the outdoor field wear strong glasses. Not that eyeglasses are not and cannot be worn successfully for sports; one purpose of this book is to show how this can be done. But in many cases, the need to wear corrective lenses develops after the choice of career or hobby, not before.

Youngsters dependent upon glasses may avoid activities which put a premium on good vision, even though they see very well with them. Reasons might be the nuisance of lenses steaming up, frames sliding down, restrictions of field view through spectacles not well designed for active sports. There could be other psychological elements involved as well. All of the physical reasons, and most of the psychological ones, can be nullified by modern visual science and thus it is possible for every youngster to enjoy the outdoors.

What really counts is not so much whether a visual deficiency exists, but what can be done with it. The visual skills the outdoorsman should have are described in Chapter 2 along with suggestions about how to test them. Many resources exist for the person whose vision is not up to par. And, in addition, there are ways to sharpen one's visual perception through experience. For most people, vision can be improved to some degree by exercise, as described in Chapter 4.

Individual Differences in Vision

Everyone needs glasses outdoors—at least at certain times—and that goes for people who have 20/20 vision. Don't drop the book! Listen to the reasons; read the material in the chapters which particularly apply to you. There is a great deal you should know about vision regardless of your natural ability to see outdoors.

To provide eye protection is reason enough to wear glasses in some situations. That can mean glasses made of safe, not ordinary shatterable, glass. But protection from glare of the sun is a major reason, and this need depends in some degree upon the eyes themselves. Small pupils are an asset outdoors in daytime. It is difficult to see comfortably in the bright sun with large pupils and generally sunglasses are required. Deep-set eyes are partially protected from glare, and overhanging brows shield the eyes from the sun above.

The natural pigment in the eye also determines in some degree its functional ability outdoors. Dark eyes are generally less sensitive to glare than light ones. Color of the iris is not the whole story, however. The amount of pigment in a deep internal layer of the retina is very important for it not only guards the visual cells, but it affects the rate of adaptation to light and dark. This rate depends upon metabolic factors in the retinal function, and these in turn depend upon the person's intake of oxygen, his diet, age, and other overall health factors. Some eyes are "night blind" because the rate of adjustment is slow or they do not reach the average level of sensitivity.

Individual differences in the optical elements of the eyes—the cornea (the clear front surface) and the crystalline lens (the small lens structure inside the eye)—mean that the effects of the harmful

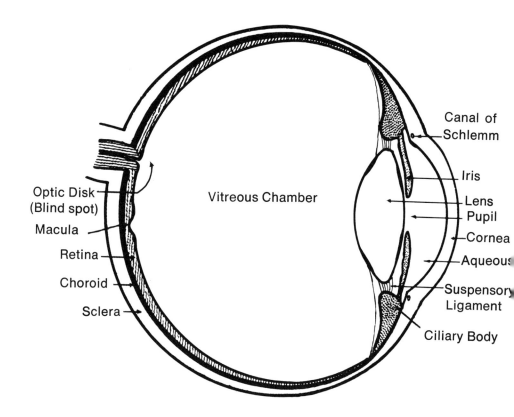

Cross-section of the human eye.

ultraviolet and infrared rays may be greater in some eyes than others. For example, there is a fluorescing effect in the crystalline lens of some eyes which can reduce good imagery. Or, the cornea and lens of the eye may not be perfect in uniformity or clarity, affecting the image and reducing visual acuity (a measure of the ability to see clearly). In such cases only limited improvement can be obtained from glasses. Such an eye is like a camera with a lens that does not transmit light perfectly.

How sharply the eye is capable of seeing also depends upon the structure of the retina and nature of the nerve elements of the visual system. Some photographic film has a fine grain while another has a coarse grain; the fine grain makes a better picture. So it is with the retina of the eye; no matter how good an image is delivered, the efficiency of reproduction depends upon anatomical factors determining its "grain" (the retinal grain).

The sensitivity and the size of the visual field can vary from one person to another. The eye is built so that it produces clear vision only in the center of its field. Visual acuity drops off drastically in the periphery. Try looking just a few degrees to one side of a test letter and you will find you cannot identify even a large one very far from your line of sight. Side vision is especially important in sport to spot objects, orient and identify them.

Some eyes have defective response in one of the three color systems, generally the red or green. Men are especially susceptible to such faulty color perception. The eye sees color as a result of various combinations of the three primary hues. (The pure scientist would shudder at that simple explanation but that is about the way it works.) Lack of response to one or more of these hues results in abnormal color perception, which is a physically inherited trait. It cannot be changed by diet, medicine, practice in perception, or time.

Effects of Age

Age has an effect on how sharply an eye can see. Some eyes are little affected by the passage of time while others lose their sensitivity in marked degree. Clouding of the crystalline lens, which is called cataract, occurs in many older eyes and this can reduce visual acuity. Cataract is highly variable in rate of development and in how seriously it bothers the individual in outdoor sports.

Even more common in affecting sight than cataract is retinal deterioration, which comes from several causes having to do with the circulatory system of the eye and the nourishment of the visual cells and the nerves. It can result in a slow diminution of sharp vision, or it can produce holes in the field of view and create some pretty drastic effects.

The lens inside the eye is regulated by a muscle which can alter the shape of the lens and thus change the distance for which the eye is focused. This tiny muscle does this with great precision so that when the eye is directed at an object, the lens is automatically focused for the proper distance. Not all eyes can do this equally well; age is a major factor and it is loss of this focusing function that makes lenses necessary as the eye gets older.

None of these age-induced deficiencies come from use of the eyes, and the eye of the outdoorsman probably stands up as well as any. To minimize the effects of age on the eye, good health care is recommended—diet, exercise, reduced tensions, and relaxed living. In addition, wearing necessary corrective or protective lenses is a wise precaution for the outdoorsman, even though it is not known whether doing so directly affects physical changes in the internal eye. Certainly his visual performance will be enhanced.

Memory Banks

Just as a camera "takes" a picture, the eye produces an image, but here the comparison ends. The eye ships the image in the form of nerve impulses to the visual areas of the brain, somewhat in the way the TV camera sends pictures to the transmitting station. But not even the TV station can be compared to the brain, where billions of cells function to interpret the information the eye has recorded. The brain does the seeing, not the eye. The brain operates something like a computer. Stored in it are memory traces of thousands of visual experiences. Incoming images are matched with what is on file. The better the file, the more accurate interpretation will be.

There is a huge difference in the kind of memory banks individuals have available to them. The British Columbia guide has compared rocks with rams so many times that his visual computer can do it with accuracy, while his inexperienced client may be lucky if he can tell rocks from rills, yet physically their eyes may be equal. The downhill skier can read a slope like the back of his hand, the fly fisherman gets the meaning of every current and eddy—once each of these sportsmen has acquired a good visual reference background.

There are two equally important aspects to skillful seeing performance outdoors. First, the eye has to produce the finest image it can get. A great deal can be done about this: lenses may help, so can exercise to improve eye movement and focusing skills.

But even with a perfect image on the retina, the interpretive mechanism of the brain must function properly. This is to some degree subject to control. Whether novice or professional, you probably can see better outdoors than you do. The chapters that follow tell how to go about it.

chapter 2

prime visual

skills for

outdoor sports

Good visual acuity rates as the most important requirement for accurate seeing. However, it is possible to be effective in sports without 20/20 vision. Some outdoorsmen, some athletes, are top-notch in proficiency with less than the normal eyesight. But any reduction in visual acuity represents at least a slight handicap in perception, which must be compensated in one way or another.

Visual Acuity

The term "20/20" refers to the size letters which the average eye can read twenty feet away. Such letters are ⅜ of an inch high. Most eyes are able to read 20/20 size, though lenses may be necessary to do it. If the letters must be made larger to be called correctly, the denominator of the fraction becomes bigger: for example, 20/40,

20/60, 20/100, and so on. The smaller the fraction, the larger the letter required to see it from twenty feet.

A person whose vision is 20/40 would require letters twice the size of those necessary for 20/20, while 20/100 letters would be five times as large. This does not necessarily mean that 20/100 visual acuity is five times worse than 20/20. It is worse, of course, but not in direct ratio to the fraction.

How much worse 20/100 vision is than 20/20 depends upon other factors. Visual acuity is only one of the visual skills a pair of eyes must have. It indicates only how clearly they see at a distance— it tells nothing about the fields of vision, the eye muscle action, the ability to see at a close point, or the speed of perception. Nor does it indicate how much "effort" or nervous energy may be needed to keep vision clear.

There are many cases of 20/20 vision in which seeing is neither comfortable nor effective. Many sportsmen who wear glasses have 20/20 vision without them. Headaches, fatigue, and eyestrain may result from use of eyes that see very clearly. Sharp vision is essential, perhaps the most important single visual skill needed outdoors, but it is not the only one a pair of eyes must have to be called "perfect."

Here are some ways to check how clearly you see:

1. Close one eye at a time and compare the appearance of a distant scene. Do objects look the same size, color, and equally clear with each eye?

2. Check with someone else. Can you see as many details as he does?

3. Next time in the field, notice if you can spot game, see the ball, or follow the action as well as you used to.

4. Use the letters in the illustration to test your visual acuity. At a distance of twenty feet, you should be able to see the letter E marked 20 quite easily with either eye—that is, the spaces between the bars should be visible. Check each eye alone. If you can only resolve the letter marked 100, you have about 20/100 visual acuity. If the 50 size is the best you can do, you have about 20/50.*

---

* No test in a book like this can be highly valid. Lighting and viewing conditions can never be perfectly controlled. These are demonstrations more than accurate tests. If you fail these, you may have a visual problem. But don't be overconfident if you pass. These tests are no substitute for a thorough visual analysis.

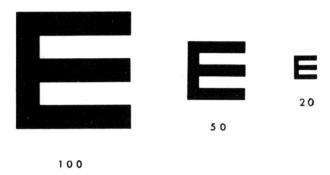

The letter marked 20 should be readable at twenty feet; to be able to do so indicates 20/20 visual acuity. If at that distance you can barely make out the one marked 50, you have 20/50 vision. If only the large letter is readable, visual acuity is 20/100.

5. Hold this book at exactly sixteen inches and see if you can read print of this size:

PROP	BELT	HERB	HERO	BURN	LONE	DOLL	DEBT	BLUE
DOME	FUEL	REED	POLE	PREY	POOL	COLT	PURE	LENS
COST	HOLY	GULF	LOVE	LEND	ROBE	BEEF	DOZY	GLEN

It takes 20/20 vision at near (the standard near testing distance is sixteen inches) to see print of this size. Move the book closer and see if you can still do it. If the print blurs after moving it only an inch or two, your near focusing power is beginning to reach the point where it may need some help.

Fields of Vision

You would not have much success if you tried walking in the woods while looking through a pair of binoculars. That tube-like viewing would greatly reduce the useful peripheral fields, and without side vision it would be very difficult to locate and orient objects even if your central vision were sharp as a tack.

Central vision is used to look directly at objects and to study their every detail. But side vision helped locate the object first, especially if it had moved, since side vision is very sensitive to motion. The whole field of view sweeps around like a radar beam to pick out a deer in a poplar grove or a flight of geese against a gray November sky.

Once an object is located, such as a landmark or a distant shore or a horseman riding on the prairie, vision is centered on it. Now binoculars are helpful to magnify the image but they are of little value in finding it in the first place.

Check your fields of vision this way: Fix your gaze on an object at eye level straight ahead. Now hold a pencil at arm's length straight out of your right, shoulder high. Can you see the end of the pencil with your side vision without shifting your gaze? If not, move the pencil forward a little until you can. Next, try the same test on your left side. Now hold the pencil above and below the fixation object in front of you. You should be able to see it at least seventy-five degrees on each side of your line of sight and about fifty degrees above and below it.

These rough demonstrations will not prove your fields of vision are normal all the time. Disease, drugs, tobacco, and alcohol can affect the visual fields. Excessive fatigue, a dead-tired condition from a day outdoors, hiking, skiing, or even fishing in rough country can reduce the sensitivity of the eye as well.

Color Vision

Spotting objects in nature against all kinds of backgrounds takes good color discrimination. The human eye has a trichromatic system. The right combination of red, green, and blue can produce all of the hue sensations the eye can see. The three primary color elements are located in the retina where they respond in appropriate intensities to the various wavelengths of light.

The color vision system never breaks down. If it is a good system to start with, color vision ability remains the same throughout life. Still, color vision deficiency is quite common. Eight percent of men, and only a fraction of one percent of women, have some degree of faulty color vision. But these people are not actually "blind" to any color. In all history, only a few hundred cases of total color blindness have been reported. In these cases, the whole color mechanism is missing, they perceive the world in black and white.

Defective color vision of the more common type results when one of the three retinal color receptors is missing or defective. Take red again for example. If the red receptor is knocked out, there is response to red wavelengths by the blue and the green receptors, but it is very weak. If the red color itself is not a bright red, or if it is seen in poor light, very little red sensation is produced in the eyes. That is about the way defective color vision works. Red objects look faded and are easily mixed up with grays and greens in so-called "red blindness." How bad the color confusion is depends upon the degree of the defect. Red and green color blindness is most common. But there are some cases of blue blindness.

About half the color-blind men have "color-weak" vision. Consider the case of red again. If the red receptor is present in the eye but just doesn't react enough, then there is a red "weakness." Reds and greens are confused only if they are similar to each other, or very dim. A person with this condition can name colors correctly; he makes only a few mistakes in distinguishing one hue from another.

There is no cure for any of the types of color blindness. Heredity is the cause and it is predominantly a male characteristic. The color system was not right in the first place. So there is no way to correct it, no way to put back the missing parts, nor to enhance the effectivity of the chemical process.

But the color-blind person is not so badly off after all. He is not really "blind." He learns to get along quite well because he finds out how to compensate for it. He may make a few mistakes in selecting neckties and be the subject of jokes by his friends, but his color-weak eyesight is no serious handicap, even outdoors.

It is even possible there is some slight advantage to having faulty color perception. The camouflage effect of birds and animals depends largely upon their colors blending with the background. But if the eye is not influenced strongly by color, the creature might be seen more easily. In wartime, color deficient observers have been used to penetrate the enemy's camouflaged emplacements.

Most important is to find out if your color perception is normal. If there is any question about your color vision, have it checked thoroughly, then learn how to compensate for any deficiency you may have.

Depth Perception

Almost every outdoor activity requires good depth judgment. Two aspects are involved—one is estimating the absolute distance to an object, the second is determining the relative distance of two objects and being able to distinguish which is closer.

There are some eight to ten clues that aid depth perception such as size, shadow, perception, and parallax. But good two-eyed seeing contributes to depth perception as well, particularly judging relative distances. An experienced one-eyed person may learn to get along quite well, but two eyes are better when they work as they should.

Poor eye-muscle coordination can prevent the two eyes from working together properly, so much so that one eye suppresses its image. Fatigue can pile up quickly when the two eyes do not function as a team. Depth perception may then become erratic as fatigue slows down normal responses; as a result attention drifts, reaction time increases. That four-pointer is away before the hunter knows it, his gun reaches his shoulder too slowly, and another beautiful miss goes down in history.

Check your own distance judgment this way:

Stand two equal-sized pencils side by side an inch apart on a table and place a book flat in front of them so that you cannot see where they touch the table. Be sure they do not cast strong shadows on the book. Move back at least fifteen feet and get your eyes level with the pencil tops.

Now close your eyes and have someone move one pencil ½ inch closer than the other. Can you judge which is closer eight times out of ten? If you are good, you should be able to discern a difference when one pencil is only ¼ inch nearer than the other.

This is only a rough illustration of ability to judge depth. It is hardly fair to call it a test. Failure would indicate inability to make gross discriminations, while success would not guarantee that depth perception is perfect. But if one eye is blurred or suppressing its image, the pencil test may detect it.

Light and Dark Adaptation

Proper adaptation to changes in light intensity is absolutely essential for outdoor sports. Brightness differences occur rapidly as one moves from deep shade to sunlight. The eye may need to guide you as you walk through the woods in the dark of night. And you may be meeting these conditions in rough and unfamiliar terrain.

Light adaptation takes place in a hurry. Even when the eye is fully adjusted to the dark, in less than a minute it can adapt to brightness almost entirely. Adaptation seems to take longer when a bright light is suddenly flashed in the eyes and they actually seem to hurt. The discomfort comes from the sudden contraction of the pupils but does not last long.

Dark adaptation takes a great deal longer and shows some variability from one person to another. About one-third of the increase in sensitivity to dim illumination occurs in the first five minutes. The process is almost complete in thirty minutes, although adaptation continues very slowly up to an hour.

The rate of dark adaptation depends upon a chemical process in the retina. This in turn is regulated by the amount of oxygen present and by vitamin A, which acts as a sort of catalyst. So diet, the state of health, and the efficiency of the eye's metabolic function are important for seeing properly at night.

There is no way you can test your dark adaptation without special equipment. Comparing with how well others see at night and how quickly they adjust to change in brightness is the best alternative. A slow response may be due to inherent physical factors. On the other hand, though rare, night blindness can be a symptom of serious eye conditions. If you no longer see in dim light as well as you used to, you should find out why.

Binocular Vision

Since there are two eyes, their images must be blended together with precision in order to get the best visual perception. The visual scientist calls seeing with two eyes *binocular vision*. If the images are not fused properly, the result can be double vision—almost worse than having only one eye. Disrupted binocular vision can lead to confused and erroneous seeing out in the field.

It takes an effective system of synchronization for the two eyes to work together properly. Each eye is aimed by six tiny muscles which attach to the outside of the eyeball. All twelve muscles of the two eyes coordinate to move the eyes so that the retinal images

are in perfect registry. This process of image blending is called
ocular fusion.

When eyes look at a distant object, the lines of sight (a line
from each eye to the object) should be parallel. They maintain this
relationship when looking to right or left, up or down, and they
must do so precisely or one eye's image will not match the other.
This is difficult for some eyes if the muscles do not function properly.
Sometimes the muscles themselves are at fault but more often it is
their nervous control.

It takes astute observation to detect eyes that do not aim and
follow objects properly and there is no good way to judge your own
performance. But by watching the eyes of another person, it is possible to detect inaccuracies in fixation as he looks from one object to
another or follows a small target moved slowly around in his field.

Fast and accurate eye movements are absolutely essential in most
sports, from skiing to skeet shooting. They can make the difference
between success and failure. In some cases, faulty eye movements
can be improved by practice. If there is any question about eye
movement skills, about the integrity of binocular vision, a thorough
visual analysis is indicated.

Besides aiming and following movements, the eyes must be able
to converge easily; meaning the two lines of sight turn inward toward
each other as they do as you read this book. If they do not converge
the right amount for the distance of the object, double vision may
be the consequence and efficiency be seriously impaired.

Hold your right forefinger out in front of you about twelve inches
from your face, and the left one out as far as you can reach. Direct
your eyes at your left finger (keep fixing it intently) and notice your
right one. You have suddenly sprouted an extra right forefinger; so
it looks anyway, if your visual response is correct and if you continue
to watch the distant object.

If you do not see the near finger double, you are suppressing vision
with one eye. With a little practice you should see two near fingers
as you fixate the farther one. If not, substitute pen flashlights for
your fingers; perhaps you can more easily see the doubled image of
the light than the extra finger.

Everything in space is always doubled except for a small area
around the object being "looked at" directly. This is true in nature
though the doubled images are so blurred they are not recognized as
being doubled. Eyes are constructed so that objects in central vision

are seen single, most others double, though you may have to look hard to find it so.

Do the "doubled finger" trick again. Now look directly at your right finger, the closer one. As your eyes aim at your right hand the two finger images should slide into one. And they should slide into one quickly; if not, your eye aiming mechanism is a bit rusty.

Now do you see a single finger on your right hand? Keep your eyes on it, and check the distant finger, on your left hand. Is it doubled? The distant finger should be doubled if your eyes are aimed properly and seeing simultaneously as they should.

Watch another person's eyes as he looks back and forth slowly from the far to near objects; notice if his eyes move smoothly and accurately. Practice until you are sure how to do it, then instruct him carefully and have him look far to near and near to far as you give the command. He should do it easily and see the doubled images as expected. Have someone watch your eyes to see if you do it correctly.

chapter **3**

visual defects
which hamper
seeing outdoors

Seeing outdoors may increase the need for visual correction—not because it aggravates defects of the eyes but rather because the sportsman in the outdoors demands good visual performance.

Symptoms of Faulty Vision

How can you tell when vision is not what it should be? Some of the ways to detect faulty vision were covered in Chapter 2. But often symptoms are vague and may not appear directly related to use of your eyes. There are always telltale signs, however, when eyesight cannot meet the demands placed on it. Here are some indicators to watch for:

Blur—One would think that blurred vision would always be easy to notice. In severe amounts it is, but in small degrees many people overlook it. Blur may develop gradually or have been present so long that the individual believes the way he sees is perfectly normal. Failure to read distant signs, squinting to see, even adjusting objects closer for a better look suggest that visual acuity is not as sharp as it should be.

Discomfort—A stinging or "pulling" sensation in the eyes or tension in head and neck muscles, sometimes extending down the back, can come from ocular disturbance. Pain or discomfort may be sharp or dull, brief or of long duration; there is no typical pattern which tells the exact cause.

Fatigue—A "my-eyes-are-tired" feeling, a general fatigue sensation of the whole body, or general listlessness, any of these can be due to eyes. This kind of fatigue may come on quickly and disappear just as fast.

Tiredness of the eyes may show up as a stiff feeling of the eyelids. The rate of blinking may speed up. Sleepiness may set in. You may want to quit whatever you are doing, even your outdoor sport becomes boring and dull, and you feel like giving your eyes a rest.

Headache—Headache which comes on after, or during, use of eyes for any critical seeing often has a visual basis. It may take only a few minutes, or it may be hours before the headache sets in. Once a headache from eyestrain has started, it may last for a long time. Rest usually stops it, so may aspirin; but it can last for days. A headache which comes on without intense eye usage, or during the night, probably has some other basis.

Nervousness—People who wear glasses often find the first sign of need for a change in prescription is an uncertain annoyance from their glasses. They pull on the frame, twist the lenses, and worry with them in general.

General nervous tension may increase. Irritability and maladjustment are hard to measure; besides much more than vision plays a part. But when these symptoms develop and no other reasons can be found, struggling eyesight may be the cause.

Double Vision—The preliminary stage to seeing double may be pulling or drawing of the eyes. This is caused by faulty muscle response. So is inability to aim and fixate objects with precision. When two images appear, something is obviously wrong and immediate attention may be necessary.

Slowing down and errors in seeing—Your boat scrapes the dock when you didn't expect it; on a downhill ski run you hit a bump that you didn't think was there; your score drops on the pistol range; or the sights of your rifle don't seem to be lined up as they should. Any drop in your usual performance when there are no other visual symptoms could be from eyesight. Do not blame it on age or lack of practice until you are sure there is no other reason.

Astigmatism

Most eyes have some astigmatism. Whether or not it creates difficulty for seeing outdoors depends upon the amount and upon how critical the need to see exactly. Riding in a boat as a passenger, you might not need a correction for moderate astigmatism, while the skipper scanning the lake for deadheads would definitely require it.

To make a good image any optical system—a camera, a telescope, or the human eye—must have light-receiving surfaces with regular

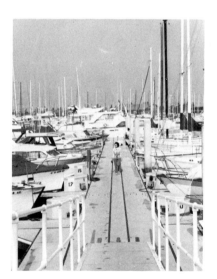 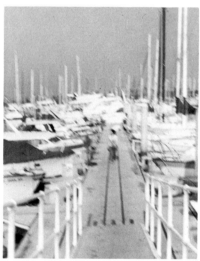

Left: Appearance of scene with normal vision.
Right: Same scene viewed with high degree of astigmatism. Notice how lines slanting diagonally down from left to right are stretched out and are almost sharp. The blur is the greatest on the diagonal down from right to left.

curvature in all meridians. If it is flat or has a different surface curvature in any of its meridians, though it may be properly curved in others, the optical system has astigmatism.

Irregularities in the shape or curvature of the human cornea produce astigmatism. The crystalline lens inside the eye is subject to the same kind of defective optical construction, though to a lesser degree. Since astigmatism is due to the physical construction of the eye, it is present early in life and remains relatively constant, changes occurring generally only over long periods of time.

Astigmatism is corrected by a lens ground with its surface curves selected to compensate for the irregularity of the major curves of the eye's refractive system. This requires that the lens be placed at an exact angle in front of the eye. A slight twist or tilt of the lens can reduce the effectiveness of the correction.

Astigmatism can cause blur or any of the discomfort symptoms. Even though visual acuity is not severely affected, it can create distortion and disorientation effects. Large degrees of astigmatism generally produce seeing difficulties that can hardly escape notice. However, the person with a small amount of astigmatism may not realize what the trouble is.

If you have astigmatism, your lenses should be kept in precise adjustment. This is especially important in the outdoors where fast action can easily get glasses out of line. This is more significant, the stronger the power. If the lens is not in proper position, it can blur vision or give a curious distorted appearance to your environment. This distortion is most evident in wide open spaces, and might not even be noticed inside a building.

Nearsightedness

Some 20 percent of outdoorsmen are nearsighted. The scientific term for nearsightedness is *myopia*. Its common name tells exactly what it is, *near vision*. It is sometimes called shortsightedness (thus, the opposite of farsightedness). The myopic eye is blurred for distance seeing, although near objects may be perfectly clear. The result is like using a camera focused for an object five feet away to take a picture of a distant scene. A blurry picture is the result.

Nearsightedness has been attributed to heredity, improper diet, endocrine imbalance, body posture, eyeball growth, or use of the

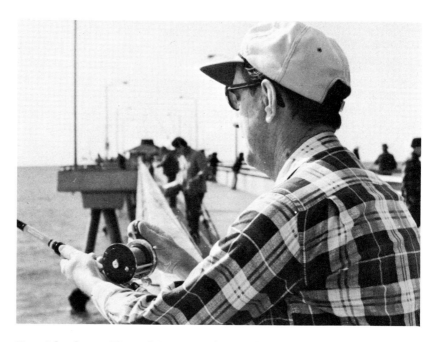

Nearsightedness. Close objects are clear and distant ones are increasingly blurred.

eyes for close work. There is no agreement as to the basic cause; in some cases all play a part. Many studies strongly suggest schoolwork causes nearsightedness.

Once the adolescent variety of nearsightedness has started, it sometimes progresses in alarming degrees. Vision continues to blur and stronger lenses are necessary at short intervals. Past the age of twenty these changes tend to decrease in frequency, and during adult life, nearsightedness is relatively stable. The outdoorsman would experience increased difficulty in seeing distant objects, even with his glasses on, if nearsightedness increased.

If eye usage is a factor in producing myopia (and this is by no means certain), it would be that which involves the eye in near seeing, not distant tasks. So outdoor use of distance vision is not a factor in producing the condition. There need be no fear then of wearing full lens corrections or "straining to see" distant objects.

Age is myopia's natural enemy. As the years roll on, the tendency is for the eyes to become less nearsighted (or more farsighted as the case may be). Vision without glasses will actually improve for the myopic eye, though usually not enough to do much practical good. However, in a very mild case, it is possible that lenses might no longer be required for distance seeing; while weaker lenses are sometimes prescribed in the later years in cases of myopia.

But myopia can show up in later life. Many times after the age of sixty, nearsightedness develops almost overnight. This may produce so-called "second sight." After wearing glasses for many years, a person can suddenly read the newspaper without them. This is caused by nearsightedness, which comes from a swelling of the lens of the eye; this puts it in focus for reading. This "second sight" is not as good as it sounds. It is produced by early cataract, a condition that also blurs distance vision.

Myopia has some good points. It seldom causes the annoying discomfort and eyestrain so common with other visual problems. It may be possible for some nearsighted persons to read comfortably without spectacles even in middle age.

Concave lenses (minus lenses) are used to compensate for the myopic eye. It is an eye that is too strong so its image focuses in front of the retina. Minus lenses are thin in the middle, thick at the edge. Because of the thinness, particularly in strong powers, they are more likely to break.

Another inconvenience is appearance and weight. In the large size lenses used outdoors, concave lenses become heavy and thick at the edge. A special kind of lens grinding may be needed to keep down the weight and improve appearances. This also suggests that the person with strong myopia should wear small glasses, unless they restrict his field of view.

Lenses for nearsightedness should be made of plastic for safety, and for reduced weight in stronger powers. And since strong concave lenses also tend to produce many annoying reflections—more so than other kinds of lenses—lens coating is especially recommended. Also, because the edges may be thick, a frame should be selected to mask the edge and improve appearance.

Presbyopia

Glasses eventually become necessary for everyone because of sagging focusing ability. Women are usually affected a few years earlier than men. The first sign is when vision becomes difficult for close work such as reading a map, telling time on a wristwatch, checking a camera setting, or any seeing within arm's length. "Longer arms or glasses" become necessary. As the condition gets progressively worse, small print blurs, eyes hurt and tire, or fatigue sets in after using the eyes only a short time.

The process which brings on this loss of near vision is technically known as *presbyopia*. It is going on in all eyes whether they are farsighted, nearsighted, have astigmatism, or are perfectly normal. Presbyopia is a progressive loss of ability to focus automatically. This reduction in focus power begins at the age of ten. From that time on, the eyes perform less efficiently in adjusting for close vision. However, they have a huge reserve power, and so trouble does not arise until reduced focusing power begins to interfere with working, reading, or seeing for an outdoor hobby.

The loss of near vision is not a development of modern civilization. It is due to the aging process, a normal physiological change in the structure of the eye. Actually the very first glasses ever used were worn to restore near vision in old people, some seven hundred years ago. Certainly using eyes for sport does nothing to aggravate the condition.

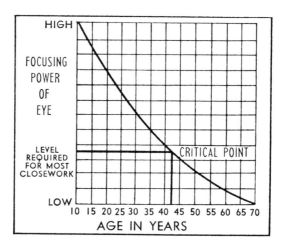

Focusing power of the eye declines with age, as illustrated by this graph. *(Courtesy of the Vision Conservation Institute)*

The loss of near vision is normal for everyone. The tiny crystalline lens of the human eye varies its shape and this is how it focuses for different distances. This lens becomes less flexible as it gets older, actually hardening so it cannot adjust as easily for a close object. Fuzzy images and eye fatigue result.

There is no known method to prevent the development of presbyopia. It may be related to the general health of the individual but no direct treatment for it is known. Proper diet and good hygiene are the only possible deterrents.

This whole process of failing near vision means that everyone in his or her forties or fifties needs glasses, and many need them long before that age. That may seem like a strong statement, but it is based on fact. Presbyopia is corrected by convex lenses, usually in the form of bifocals, to aid the eye focus.

By no means does every outdoorsman have to be chained permanently to spectacles. The demand on near vision for sports is relatively mild in most cases. When a problem does deevlop, the solution is complex because of the importance of sharp distance vision and the need of the wearer to walk and move around a great deal. Lens designs for individual sports are discussed later in this book. But for the best possible vision for both distance and near, few eyes can do without some help as age sneaks up.

The moment you read that, you will probably think of an exception. Your Uncle Harry, or your neighbor's grandmother perhaps, could "read the newspaper without glasses." But was this really an exception to the rule?

True, some people past age fifty can read without glasses. Maybe the "reading" involved only looking at the headlines. Or perhaps the person was slightly nearsighted and could see within arm's length quite well.

But when the older person can read without glasses, the chances are his distance vision is not clear and he no longer has 20/20. He may not realize this; possibly he does not drive or encounter more than casual demands on his sight. Regardless of what the individual might *think* about his own visual performance, even though he is quite satisfied with it, a thorough examination would reveal he does not see perfectly once he has reached "middle age."

There is one possible exception. The person with one eye which is nearsighted just the right amount can read nicely with it; then if the other is slightly farsighted, he can use it for distance seeing. This handy arrangement provides both near and far vision without glasses, though only one eye is used at a time. It takes a lucky combination of circumstances and it is extremely rare to have good vision at all distances once age fifty has been passed.

Some day, glasses will be needed even more than they are now if you are farsighted. It's inevitable. That's the annoying characteristic of farsightedness as the compensating focusing ability gets progressively less as time goes on. The sportsman in later life, though never troubled before, may find his distance vision blurs and that he needs to wear glasses to improve his outdoor visual performance.

Farsightedness

Many people who wear glasses can see clearly without them. This is true of many farsighted eyes and could lead to the belief that glasses are not necessary for use in the outdoors. The degree of far-sightedness and the vision requirement of the outdoor activity determine whether or not this is true. The farsighted eye is truly a "far seeing eye." Technically, the condition is called *hyperopia* and it is more or less troublesome, depending on how effectively the eye is able to focus and compensate.

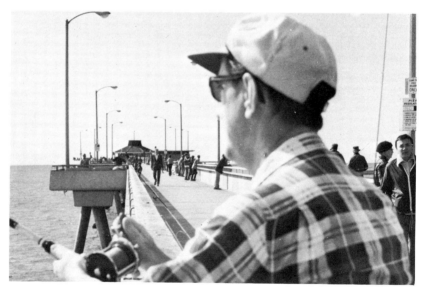

Farsightedness. Distant objects are sharp and clear but those nearby are blurred.

The hyperopic eye is built in such a way that when the little internal eye muscle controlling the lens is completely relaxed, the eye is out of focus. The farsighted person must constantly maintain a little focus effort to keep clear vision. If the eye has lots of far-sightedness and only a little focus power, vision can be blurred. Even though you have perfectly sharp distance vision right now, it is quite possible that some day it will blur and you will need glasses to clear it up.

The eyes of most infants are quite farsighted: 80 to 90 percent are found to be so in the first few years of life. As the eyes grow and develop this condition diminishes until in the early teens only a small amount is left. It is considered normal to be slightly farsighted in the twenties and thirties. Then at about age forty, hyperopia begins slowly to increase. At some point after this the farsighted eye becomes troublesome, depending upon how much strain is put on it and how much focus power is left.

It is true that mild amounts of farsightedness may not require correcting for casual outdoor seeing. The hunter, the marksman, the flyer or driver may, however, have trouble trying to keep eyes in focus. Blurred vision is not a likely symptom; rather fatigue, nervousness, headache are the potential consequences.

Convex lenses (plus power lenses) are used to set the farsighted eye at rest. They do some of the focusing for the eyes, and thus knock out strain and tension. The length of time glasses need be worn depends upon how bad the farsightedness is. Sometimes they are required only when the eyes are used intently. If vision is blurred without them or the amount of eyestrain is great, spectacles will probably have to be worn full time. Plus lenses are thick in the center, thin at the edge. They tend to be safer than concave lenses, though lenses worn outdoors should always be break-resistant or plastic. In strong powers, they are very heavy in glass. Reflections are not especially bad but coating is generally beneficial. Since edges are thin, they must fit the frame edge perfectly to prevent chipping.

You can use your eyes all you want to and have no fear it will bring on presbyopia. Eyes can't be worn out or damaged by using them if they receive visual care when necessary. No need to make yourself a visual cripple, giving up the things you like to do for sport and relaxation, in order to protect your eyesight. Certainly it should not be the end of fishing or hunting days. Most important is early correction with glasses and frequent care as the need arises—these measures can provide continuous, productive seeing, free from discomfort and worry.

Eye Muscle Problems

Visual training can sometimes remedy the inability to move and fixate the two eyes properly or to coordinate them so that the two retinal images register perfectly on each eye. This is discussed in Chapter 2. But there are muscle balance problems which can be corrected by lenses.

Sometimes the tone of the muscles which control the eyes is such that one eye tends to turn up or down, in or out, a little too much. At least it is the same as if this were the case. A properly prescribed prism lens is sometimes used to relieve this condition.

A prism bends light without changing its focus. This makes it possible for the eye to assume the posture dictated by its muscle tone yet to have the image placed on its retina in the proper position. A prism is selected of the appropriate power to bend the light to do this. A prism lens is thicker on one edge than the opposite, though the difference is slight in weaker powers.

Correction is important for the sportsman because ocular muscle imbalance may cause fatigue and make seeing difficult, especially if the imbalance is in the vertical direction. The symptoms of the problem are discomfort, and inefficiency, never blur; though in marked imbalances, double vision can occur. Fortunately, correction is rather easy and should be done for every sportsman with significant muscle imbalance whose visual mechanism is placed in stress.

Glasses Don't Ruin Eyesight

The rugged outdoorsman may disdain wearing glasses thinking they will "ruin" his eyes. He is mistaken. Sometimes it seems as if lenses make eyesight weaker. The reason is that it is no fun to go without glasses after enjoying the good seeing they produce. Uncorrected vision may even appear more blurry than it did before glasses, but the lenses were not the cause; the blur was there and eventually would have been noticed.

Often this wrong idea about seeing develops when a person in the forty-plus age first puts on glasses. Close vision is naturally getting harder along about this time, and since it appears to do so all of a sudden, spectacles sometimes get the blame because it is no longer possible to read without them.

The greatest preventive against "ruining eyesight" at any age is getting professional care when it is first needed. Postponement jeopardizes comfort, efficiency, and even one's safety. Once vision gets too far behind, it is hard to bring it back to par. You cannot keep your eyes strong and healthy by "not giving in to glasses.". You are taking unnecessary chances if you neglect your precious eyesight by doing that.

Glasses are one reason the modern sportsman is so much better than his ancestors. Half of Sitting Bull's war party may have had miserable visual acuity and never knew, or could not have corrected it if they did. Or perhaps those who had bad vision were left in camp with the squaws. Such a fate need never befall anyone today.

chapter 4

how to see

even better

outdoors

Eyesight for sport can be improved to some degree by practice and by applying some fundamentals of visual perception. Even the expert can increase his perceptual abilities, while the novice could conceivably learn to read nature like an Alaskan backwoodsman. With top quality visual performance everyone has a lot to gain in sheer enjoyment of the outdoors.

First of all, the eye should have the finest visual acuity it can get. The retina needs the best possible image if it is to do an accurate job of reporting about the outside world. Defects of vision which should be corrected have been described in the preceding chapter. Generally, any lens prescription for distance seeing should be worn in the outdoors.

Sharpening Perceptual Skills

But even with a sharp image, interpreting what a blob of light and dark and color means takes a lot of perceptual skill—skill that is not automatically the same for each person. The farmer can find a rabbit in a fence row quicker than anyone else because he has had a lot of practice; so his visual perception is actually sharper in the field.

The man who hunts once a year can never reach a state of visual perfection from experience in the field alone, even if he lives to the age of one hundred and fifty. But anyone can practice improving his visual acuity and he can do it every day. Within certain limits the eye can be taught to get more meaning out of an image on its retina; or, more correctly, the brain can learn to make more sense of what the eye sees.

Practice while walking, or driving, or relaxing, as long as you are not jeopardizing your comfort or safety. Try to recognize objects as far away as you can and resolve their details. Attempt to read signs before you think you really can. Work diligently at trying to sharpen your sight every time you are in the field—look at the trees, not the forest. If you are serious, practice at home with small objects or cut-out letters at a great distance.

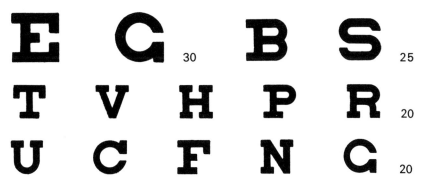

Practice reading these letters from as far away as you can. Numbers at the side indicate distance in feet from which they should normally be visible.

A good practice device is a block E about an inch high on a white circle. Have someone rotate the circle so that from your observation distance you can not see which way the letter opens. Move forward until you can just make it out. Work backward as far as possible. Do this five minutes a day.

If you work at sharpening your perception, you will learn one of the secrets of the expert. He can locate objects he can not really see!

It has been shown in laboratory experiments that when trained observers are forced to name letters that they *say* are too small to make out they call them correctly a high percentage of the time. Try this in the field. Attempt to name and identify objects even before you are sure what they are.

Keep Eyes Moving

Try staring steadily at a small distant object. Hold on it for five minutes. Your eyes may begin to water, the object will probably blur, and it will be difficult to stay still as a sense of discomfort builds up. Steady fixation violates a fundamental rule of good seeing: keep your eyes moving.

It is a natural tendency of eye muscles to make the eye rove. If they hold steady very long, fatigue develops quickly and their efficiency drops. Only a tiny fraction of the muscle fibers of the eye muscles operate at any one time but they need to rest frequently. The whole system is refreshed if movements are made to shift the tension from one set of fibers to another.

Another good reason for constantly moving the eyes is to prevent too much adaptation to things as they are. The eye tends to lose its sensitivity to a fixed image on the retina. Many a marksman has experienced this: Staring at a bull's-eye they find that it suddenly disappears. This can happen if you fix too long on a motionless figure. Move your eyes to maintain their sensitivity.

The sweeping process should be fast and accurate. Scan the whole field carefully. Stop. Evaluate all you see quickly, then move on. Practice it every time you are outdoors. Move, blink, look at one object then another; let it become automatic.

If your eye movements are sluggish, build them with some home exercises. Roll your eyes slowly in circles with lids closed, then open. Holding your head still, glance to the corners of the room. Try it on the ceiling while lying in bed. In a sitting position, select objects on the wall, look rhythmically from one to the other, reverse direction.

These exercises can be beneficial after, or during, a long day in the field to relax the eyes. Move your eyes slowly and regularly in large circles. Then see how many objects in the field of view you can fixate accurately in thirty seconds. Stop for fifteen seconds then repeat.

Perceptive Set

Knowledge of the outdoors, of the habits of animals, of the meaning of nature's signs can help a great deal in perceiving. But knowledge and experience are not everything. Some fundamental perceiving skills can be made to work better if you know how.

Study the habits of game and of fish to aid you in the field. Even knowledge of the terrain, the trees, and plants, is useful; the sky, the shoreline, the contour of the road and whatever else comes into view in an outdoor sport are part of the reference background that aids seeing accuracy. The person who spends fifty weeks a year looking at four walls of an office probably knows next to nothing about antlered animals' forage plants. Yet, if he did, he would know where he might find a moose.

Now there is nothing startling about the suggestion to know the inside and out of a sport. Every sportsman has heard it. But the chances are that he does not know how to develop the proper seeing attitude. The visual scientist calls this "perceptive set," a quality that has been found to be very effective in training subjects to see better.

A difference in perceptive set explains why one individual can spot objects quicker than another. The fisherman does not consciously decide to turn on his perceptive set when he is looking for the distant riffle of a school of bait fish. Yet he gets ready to react. The skeet shooter shows this very clearly as he crouches forward before each clay bird release.

"Set" is alertness, being ready for anything with confidence. It is a certain "I'm ready" attitude that makes the laws of seeing in the field go to work better. It is the batter getting set to see the pitcher's blinding fast ball. It is the botanist's sense of readiness to pick out the leaves of a rare plant amidst a mass of foliage.

You can develop the proper set for seeing better. You need not strain to see, nor should you relax completely. Rather, you adopt an attitude between those extremes—the entire body and all the senses, not just vision, get ready to react to what is going on. You are in a condition of total relaxed alertness.

To sharpen your perceptive skill clear your mind of problems. Think about perceiving *sounds* as well as visual images. Practice identifying the makes of cars as accurately as you can in a brief glance. In a park or other outdoor area, walk a hundred yards then stop and recall all the different things you saw.

Here are some other suggestions which can help. Try to see things for the purpose of *remembering,* which is different than just looking. Use the association method, relate things to each other. Right after an experience, *work* at retention; recount what you saw.

Speed of Recognition

How long would it take you to memorize the number 728395410-862? Could you do it in a fraction of a second?

The eye can see well enough to grasp the twelve numbers, but the mind needs time to learn them. Using an instrument which has the peculiar name of tachistoscope, it is possible to train the speed of recognition. This instrument can flash letters, words, or numbers on a screen for rapid exposure times. The average eye should be able to see five numbers exposed for only 1/100 of a second.

The speed of seeing can be increased dramatically. Pictures, silhouettes, clues are flashed before the observer, who must identify them instantly. This has been done many times in laboratory situations and is a method used by the military services to enhance the ability to recognize planes, whether friend or foe.

Increasing speed of recognition is best done with a mechanical device like the tachistoscope that exposes numbers, pictures, symbols for a fraction of a second. Not worth the trouble? Well that depends upon your goal. If you want to become the champion trapshooter in your club, it might be. If perceiving outdoors is the way you earn your living, or even if it creates a good share of your fun, it might be. Seek professional advice to lay out a specific training program for your needs if you sincerely want to enhance your perceptual skills.

Some simple flashing devices are available or you can make your own. Targets can be made with line drawings, cut-outs of wildlife, number or forms, or the two-by-two-inch slides you already have. Using an ordinary projector block the lens with a card, then uncover it for an instant. Try for accurate recall. Visualize as many details as possible in each exposure. Then show the picture again to check your accuracy. Verification is a vital part of the learning process.

The span of recognition can also be enhanced with pacing devices used when reading. These force the eye to move along rather rapidly without dwelling too long on each word. How fast you read depends upon how much is taken in during each fixation and your ability to do this can be improved.

Cut a slot in a small cardboard big enough to expose a set of fixed digits. You can type the digits in columns double spaced. Place the cardboard over the columns so that no number shows in the slot. Move the slot up to expose a number for just an instant, stopping so no number shows. Try to repeat the number that flashed in the opening. Practice until you can do six and seven digits, even more.

Type or print columns to practice with. Work with as many numbers as you can get in a flash; increase the number as you improve. Slide the slot across a number. Repeat it aloud. Move the slot back to verify your accuracy. Practice of this type can increase your span of recognition and it can have carry-over value for seeing outdoors.

Optical Illusions in Nature

No matter how well your eyes work and how skillful your perception, there are some optical illusions which can fool you. One is caused by the way light is bent in going from water into air. Unless you look straight down at a right angle to the water, a fish is never where you see him. Rays of light are bent slightly toward the horizontal as they leave the water and go into the air, so a submerged object appears farther away than it really is. When casting, drop the lure a little closer to you than the fish seems to be.

An object seen through extreme contrasts of hot and cold layers of air will appear displaced from its true position. This illusion could be the cause of a missed shot at a trophy head. The effect produces certain kinds of mirages—a lake or a hilltop appearing where there is none—and such physical illusions can actually be photographed!

Seeing distortions in nature can also be a result of brightness and color differences. A tan-colored animal, for instance a deer, seen against a very dark background of trees or mountains will appear lighter than he really is. Seeming lighter, and thus brighter, he will appear closer than he is. The opposite is also true; seen against snow, he will appear darker and thus farther away.

This illusory principle can work another way too. Objects far away look larger than they really are, close objects appear smaller. The

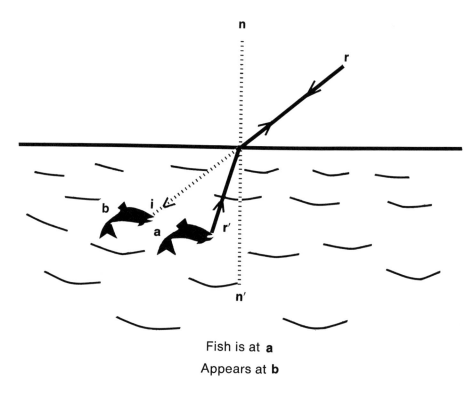

Fish is at **a**

Appears at **b**

Light from fish at a is refracted when going into air along line r. Eye looking along the refracted ray r sees the image of the fish at b. n, n' is the normal, a line perpendicular to the surface of the water. r', r is the path of light from the real fish. r, i is the path of the projected image seen by the eye.

situation is further complicated by the viewer's experience, the background, lighting, and a time factor, all of which influence illusions. A herd of antelope at 600 yards will shrink in size when you come right up on them. The famous moon illusion is a striking example of the size and distance effect. The moon always looks huge on the horizon but small at its zenith. Yet it is a constant distance away and never changes size. When photographed, it appears on the film exactly the same size in each position, even though it did not look that way to the eye.

What happens is that the human perceptual mechanism projects

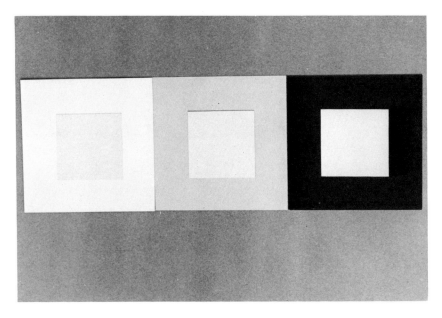

Background determines how bright an object appears to be. Here the center squares are all cut from the same piece of grey paper but they do not look the same. This principle works in nature too.

how to allow for the lighting on a long-range shot, yet he could hardly describe how if asked.

Haze creates a distance illusion. Ever notice how mountains seem closer when they are clearer? Haze, the bluish cast it creates, makes objects seem farther away than they are in reality. When it is hazy, things are actually closer than they look.

Movement illusions can fool you also. It is possible for one object to move yet the observer think the movement was made by something else. Has this ever happened to you? Sitting in an anchored boat you suddenly feel the boat has started to move. It is the waves and water surface that are actually moving. Perceptually, you and the boat become figure and the water becomes ground. Figure moves, never background.

Since there is no changing illusions in nature, what can you do about them? Understanding the principles will help you recognize when you might be fooled. Besides that, sharpening your total per-

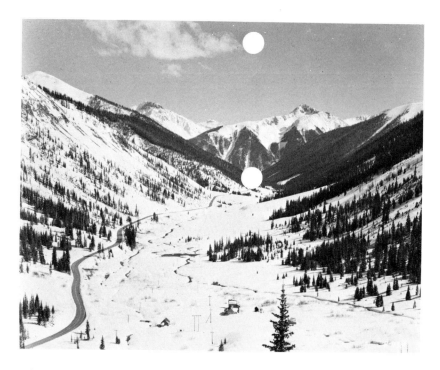

Which white spot looks larger in this Colorado mountain scene illustrating the well known moon illusion? The object appearing farther away (in this case the lower one) looks larger.

ceptive ability is a good precaution. The experienced hunter knows the moon's image is farther away on the horizon than when overhead, partly because of the "filled space" on the earth's surface (the trees, the buildings, and the objects the observer sees between himself and the horizon) and the emptiness upward. Thus, if the moon were actually farther away, it would have to be larger to create the same-sized retinal image it does from its zenith. So it actually appears larger. This principle has been proved by careful scientific experiments.

Cutting Down the Effects of Illusions

Though some illusions are always present, there are ways to minimize the effects and improve seeing accuracy:

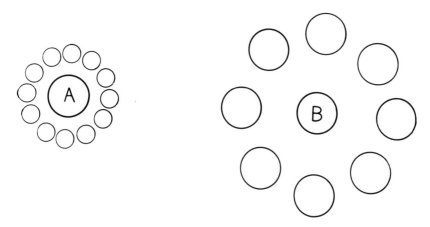

The size of an object in nature looks large or small depending on what is handy for comparison. The eye is easily fooled. Circles A and B are the same size.

1. Carry some standard distances in your head. Have your visual yardstick—a football field, the width of a room, the height of your garage. Estimate distance in terms of this standard which you can express in yards or feet. Practice estimating distance, then step it off, using your own length of stride.

2. Pin down size as accurately as you can. Known objects have a fixed size—a man, a canoe, a football. Judge their distance by their apparent size. Apply the same principles to unknown objects.

3. Compare objects with their background. A mountain lion should not look the size of a house cat because it is standing in front of a giant pine tree. Make judgments on a what-seems-logical basis.

4. Don't be fooled by brightness and color. Dim objects appear farther away than they are. Blue and dark objects also seem dim and thus far away.

5. Blurry vision, dirty glasses, sunglasses worn at night, even a rainy atmosphere all reduce the brightness of objects. This can make them seem distant and small.

6. Watch for shadow direction and overlap to tell which object is closer. Move your eyes. Fixate at different distances. Be aggressive and alert in all visual judgments.

7. Head motion will improve depth judgment. The scientist calls this motion parallax. Hold a forefinger up in front of you at arm's

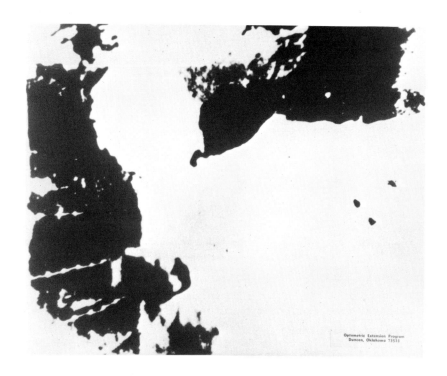

Optometric Extension Program
Duncan, Oklahoma 73533

There is an animal in this picture—one that everybody knows well. Can you see it? It is not hidden or camouflaged but occupies most of the picture. If you cannot see it, turn to page 201 for the answer. Notice that once you know what it is, it is easy to see again and again. This experiment tells a lot about seeing. Once you can make a good figure out of a mass of light and dark on the retina, it remains quite stable. (*Courtesy of the Optometric Extension Program Foundation*)

length. Hold the other one about a foot from your eyes. While you sight on the farthest one, move your head from side to side. Notice the closer finger will move opposite the direction of head movement. Distant objects move the same way as the head. Look at the near finger to check this.

Try the motion parallax effect on objects outdoors—trees, buildings, cars. It is a useful clue in judging where objects are in relation to each other. So move your head when you are sizing things up. Parallax works for you even though you are not conscious of it so you don't have to remember which moves opposite or the same, but you do have to move your head rather vigorously.

8. Be sure your eyes have plenty of time to adapt before trying to come close to maximum sensitivity. So before sailing away from the dock or hiking into the woods at night, shield your eyes from light for some time before you peer into darkness. Look from bright to dark areas rather than the reverse.

The eye is less sensitive to red with its night vision system than any other color. Thus the retina can go ahead and adapt to dark quite well even though red light is falling on it. This is the reason fighter pilots wear red glasses in the "ready" room before going on a night mission. Thirty minutes with red goggles is enough to boost the eye's sensitivity to dim light manyfold.

Simply reducing illumination wherever you are before going into the dark will allow some preadaption. Even better is wearing a red lens, if night vision is particularly critical for you. Wearing dark lenses indoors will help some since they shield the eyes somewhat (but dark lenses should never be worn indoors for any other reason).

Exposure to ordinary sunlight has been found to produce both temporary and cumulative effects on night vision. After daily exposure to bright sun without sunglasses for about ten days, one investigator found the loss in night vision corresponded to about a 50 percent deterioration in visual acuity.

Persons engaged in tasks where night vision is critical should wear sunglasses when in bright sunlight. (See Chapter 9, which discusses sunglasses.) Boat and plane pilots, even auto drivers in some circumstances, benefit from protecting the night vision mechanism from too much sun during the day.

Another trick to spot a dim object at night is to look just a little to the side of where you expect it to be. This causes its image to fall on the area of the retina most sensitive to weak light. Try it with a faint star: look about five degrees to either side and it will appear brighter if your eyes are thoroughly dark adapted.

Seeing with Faulty Color Vision

There is no way to improve color vision that is normal. Practice and learning have little or no effect on hue discrimination ability. However, the suggestions which follow apply to making any color judgments. But with faulty color vision, there are effective ways to reduce potential seeing errors:

1. Be careful in dim light, early in the morning and in twilight. Errors in discrimination are most likely when objects are dim or small.
2. Watch reds and greens. These colors are most likely to be confused.
3. Look for differences in brightness rather than hue.
4. Take time to make judgments.
5. Make comparisons with known objects and colors when you can.

Being Seen in the Outdoors

Hunting is the obvious case in which it is wise to be highly visible to other hunters. This can be done by wearing certain bright colors which are not visible to game animals (see the following chapter, which discusses vision of animals). There might be other times when being readily seen is highly desirable—hiking, exploring, or around the water.

The color which is most visible depends upon the function of the human eye. Though red was long used as a "safe" color, it is exactly the opposite. Red is the color to which the eye is least sensitive. It fades to black or brown in dim light and also looks very much like fall foliage. For this reason alone, it could be dangerous to wear in early morning or twilight.

Another reason red is a poor choice for a "safe" color is that it is the color which a large number of male eyes see very poorly. The color-deficient eye can see almost any color better than red. So strolling in the field in a red coat is a bit risky, since one out of every twelve hunters has some difficulty seeing red.

The eye is the most sensitive to the middle of the spectrum, the yellows and oranges. These colors have much higher visibility and have been proven so in field tests. There have been slight differences in results of several research groups but blaze orange and yellow come out to be the winners. Extensive field tests conducted in California to determine which color was most visible, led to the conclusion that yellow had the highest visibility. The studies were done in a number of locales and with a number of subjects, some of whom were color deficient. The results indicated that a yellow had very high visibility—though it does tend to look like white.

Additional field tests made in Massachusetts proved that a blaze orange color was even superior for high visibility. Under some conditions, yellow looked white and could be mistaken for a whitetailed deer. Blaze orange does not look like anything else in nature and therefore is obviously "man-made." It has now been widely accepted as the safest color for hunters to wear.

The hunter who wears drab colors, olive or brown, is taking a big chance. Deer hunting is the most dangerous for there are usually lots of hunters moving in wooded country. Man resembles the size of a deer, stands about the same height. In dim light, it is not hard for an anxious hunter to conjure up a deer where there is none.

Man's visual perception can be fooled. Straining to see in early dawn can put stumps and branches together to make a deer. In fact, starting in very poor seeing conditions may prolong the ability to resolve fuzzy shadows into real objects. With only a few clues, and wanting so badly to spot game, the hunter may imagine that a movement, a flash of white, and a shadow of brown means a trophy buck.

That is why it is so important to wear blaze orange. A fluorescent color never belonged to any game animal and it calls a halt to those suggestive clues that could turn man into a target and lead to a tragic mistake.

"Tension Relievers"

Fatigue can be an enemy of good vision, and it may be beneficial to rest and relax your eyes if you feel fatigue setting in.

Listed below are some "tension relievers." They are not exercises to strengthen your eyes or to get rid of spectacles, and above all, they are not substitutes for visual care. Never attempt to diagnose your own visual problems. Do these exercises only if you are sure you have no visual problem which needs correction.

1. Glance around to the extreme corners of the room without moving your head. Look slowly and rhythmically from one spot to another.

2. After a minute or two of the fixational movements, close your eyes and rest for ten seconds, blink a few times, then rest for ten seconds more.

3. Repeat the looking-around-the-room movements in the opposite

direction, rapidly for fifteen seconds. Then close your eyes and count slowly to twenty.

This simple routine may be enough to eliminate mild fatigue. If not, repeat several times or add the following rotational exercises:

1. Roll your eyes in large circles for thirty seconds, reverse direction for another thirty seconds.

2. Close your eyes to rest for ten seconds, blink a few times.

3. Now fixate a spot on the distant wall; keep your eyes on it while you roll your head around first one way, then the other. Thirty seconds in each direction will do.

4. Lean back in your chair and relax a few minutes doing nothing.

chapter 5

how animals

see

You are perfectly safe waving a red flag at Farmer John's ferocious bull—at least the color makes no difference! Bulls do not have color vision. The fluttering cloth might incite the bull to charge, but any color would do the same. The world is seen in shades of black and white by all color-blind creatures. And this includes most of the animals man has domesticated, along with many that roam free.

The "eyes" of some simple forms of life are merely small bunches of light-sensitive cells. These nerve spots can do nothing but detect the presence of light and roughly judge its brightness. They may guide the creature to warmth or food or may lead it from harm. Even these "simple" eyes have their purpose, as do all the wide variety of eyes found in nature's realm.

Birds, noted for their sharp vision, can fly through the branches of a tree at top speed. Their excellent color vision enables them to penetrate their prey's cleverest camouflage. Hawks and eagles have vision that is four to eight times sharper than man's, while many birds can focus forty times as much and ten times as fast.

Because birds can see color, they are best approached by wearing clothes which blend with the surroundings. However, they can also readily detect motion and it takes careful stalking to get close to them. In addition, most of the birds which are prey to many predators, including the song birds, have eyes at the sides of their heads; so they are endowed with a wide field of vision to look for enemies. It is not easy to sneak up on an alert bird that can see in a very broad field.

The predatory "hunters," the meat-eating birds, have their eyes in the front of their heads, where the fields of vision of each eye overlap; though reducing their total field of view, this arrangement enables them to locate prey quickly and accurately. Since their field is small, it is possible to come up behind them without being seen.

The two eyes of some birds weigh more than their brains and their eyeballs are larger than man's. Their retinas have lots of cone cells which permit sharp vision. But for all their keen eyesight, most birds are blinded in dim light and their feeble brains understand but little of the world about them. The exceptions are the owls. They have retinas with an immense number of rods—the visual cells adapted to see in dim light. Their eyes are built quite differently from those of their diurnal relatives. Even the pupils open much wider and have a different shape.

Possum, raccoon, certain fish which live in the ocean depths, and the other night prowlers have eyes specialized for seeing in dim light. The retinas of their eyes are also packed with super-sensitive cells which react quickly to the very feeble light. They can best be approached in complete darkness; once discovered, however, they may be "blinded" by light directly in their eyes.

Monkeys have vision most like that of man. They have eyes which are built and function in a similar way and they can see in both day and night. Some monkeys even seem to be subject to the same types of defective color vision.

More is being learned all the time about the vision of insects. Bees and many fast-flying insects can see things invisible to humans because their eyes are sensitive to certain wavelengths of light that are very short. Insects can apparently distinguish moving objects very easily. Many have compound eyes with thousands of tiny lenses. (No one has yet figured out how to make the outdoorsman "invisible" to avoid the biting varieties.)

Reptiles and lizards are thought to have some color vision but even more interesting are their built-in safety goggles. Tough protective coverings keep their eyes shielded from sand and dirt. These transparent eyelids enable them to go right on seeing without injury to the sensitive interior of the eye. But they have no eylids to close and must sleep with their eyes open.

All of America's game animals are color-blind. A hunter's jacket of blaze orange, or any color for that matter, may seem to a deer, elk, bear or similar animal to blend perfectly into the wooded background. They rely on smell and movement far more than eyesight to detect danger. Game animals probably do not have nearly as good visual acuity as man. A few, such as the rhino, have notoriously poor eyesight. But all can detect movement easily. It is doubtful if wild animals know the shape of a man. His behavior probably worries them as much as his form.

Even man's best friend, the dog, is color-blind. It makes no difference to the hound if his quarry is the same color as the bush which hides it. He too depends mainly on smell and movement, and he may not "see" a motionless rabbit in plain sight. But the hunting dog may be able to get more sensations out of black and white alone than man who has color to help him see.

The cat, and most of his relatives, live in a drab colorless world. He has superior eyesight at night and he can get by in the daytime, although his vision is only one sixth as sharp as the human eye. Yet members of the cat family such as lions and tigers can hunt in the daytime. Their centrally placed eyes enable them to follow and pursue running prey.

The fisherman dangling his bait close in front of a fish's nose is wasting his time. There is a completely blind zone in front of a fish, and bait can be seen only if it is farther away or off to one side. Game fish with skeletons of bone, like bass and trout, have color vision. They can be attracted by bright colored lures.

Why certain color lures work one time and not another no one knows. But they do. Perhaps it is a combination of color against the background that excites a fish to strike. One color works in one lake, one in another and even differences in seasons play a part. But if the fish are not biting try changing lures; you can never tell what color might be the fishes' favorite of the day.

There is very little experimental evidence about fishes' color vision, particularly those which pose a threat to a diver. But known facts about anatomy, histology, and visual function permit some assumptions. With regard to eyesight, a sharp line appears to be drawn between fish which have skeletons of cartilage (the elasmobranches), which includes all the shark and rays, and all the rest of the fish which have skeletons of bone (the teleosts).

It seems quite certain that the shark and rays do not have color vision; indeed, they have very dim eyesight. Thus it makes no difference to a shark what color a diver is, although he will perceive how *bright* he appears to be. However, it takes more than brightness to invite attack. Smell, possibly, type of movement (simulating action of fish), depth, location, and perhaps other factors that are as yet unknown, all play a part.

Pattern rather than *color* may well be a factor in attracting fish. Scientific study has not yet determined if this is so. From what is known you might assume that if you do not want a shark to see you, you should use dark clothes and equipment. This does not mean that if a shark does see you, he will attack, nor that he will not attack when he cannot see you. Too few facts are available to accurately weigh how much the shark's eyesight affects his inclination to attack.

Fish other than sharks and rays apparently do have color vision. They may be attracted by color or frightened away by it. Color which stands out from the prevailing surroundings might be highly visible to them. Barracuda, for example, are attracted by bright-colored objects. This fish also has a type of eye which gives sharper vision than that of the shark. So it seems that barracuda and other bony fish can better decide visually what a thing is. It is possible that the right color, or pattern of colors, might ward them off—but this is only a guess.

The more the diver looks like a fish, the more he invites investigation by predators. The more inconspicuous he is, the less likely to attract notice, the more easily he may be confused with fish. There are times when fish seem to feed and strike at anything, even a bare hook, which at other times may frighten them away, but much more is involved than visual appearance alone.

Though a dark suit may hide the diver from fish, it certainly makes him less visible to his buddies. In case of emergency, the brightest possible color on you and on your equipment could save your life. A pattern or stripe that is different from anything found in the sea would also enhance visibility.

Science must provide the answer as to what color is best for visibility in water. Whether the golden-yellow to orange-yellow range is best under water as well as on land is not certain, although it seems logical it would be. Again, red is the color that fades out first in water (and so would a red object which looks "red" because it reflects red light).

Yellow holds down to 300 feet in depth; beyond that, blue penetrates better and perhaps blue colors would be visible. On the other hand, blue would blend easily with the undersea background. Beyond 300 feet, however, color may make little difference because the amount of light is very low and the eye does not see color in true night vision. White may well be the best choice to reflect all available light at great depths.

to fish, and at the same time hard for other divers to see, or to increase visibility for your buddies, and assume fish are little concerned with color. The choice should be considered in terms of the kind of diving done, the conditions in which it is done, fish found in the area, and of course the type of equipment which is used.

Animals' eyes are built in ingenious ways to accomplish their special purpose. Some have large retinas, small lenses, slit-like pupils, tilted eyes, even shiny surfaces to reflect light back for better seeing, like the eyes of a cat which shine in the dark. The creatures which travel chiefly at night have eyes adapted well to dim light. Those which move around mostly by day have sharp eyesight in bright illumination and usually have color vision to go along with it. And there are many other ways eyes are specialized to do a particular job.

Eyes are even placed in the head in such a way to be most useful. Some fish have eyes at the top of their skulls to look up into the air above from whence danger might come. Certain birds can see downward without moving their heads, another handy safety device. Animals and birds which are common prey of many predators have eyes at the side of their heads, which gives them a wide field of view to look for potential enemies. The hunters, the predators in nature's realm, have eyes in the front of their skulls where the overlapping visual fields can help locate prey quickly and accurately.

The question really is whether to be as inconspicuous as possible

Whatever eyesight a creature possesses, good or bad according to man's standard, it serves *him* well. His habits, his very life depend upon his vision, whether he has a simple "spot" for an eye, or a complete visual apparatus with millions of elaborate nerve cells. Even the lowly mole needs eyesight, and he has enough to "see" light showing through the broken burrow when it needs repairing.

Man has the finest eyesight of all. Some animals can see more sharply, many can see better at night, but none can operate as effectively in such a wide range of environments. Animals with vision superior to man's in some ways, often have eyes hooked to small and sluggish brains. Man has a dual-purpose eye for seeing both day and night, and it pours information into a vastly superior brain.

part **two**

aids to
better
vision

chapter **6**

corrective and
safety lenses

When most people have their vision examined they tell about visual symptoms and how they use their eyes at work. This is as it should be. However, it does not follow that a lens prescription designed for office, factory, or farm is necessarily correct for outdoor sports.

Do you water ski, play golf, shoot with a bow for distance, or drive a sports car? Which outdoor activity or activities you go in for can make a difference in your lens prescription, and in many of its details, such as kind of lens, tint, size, and location of optical centers. There is also the whole question of whether a multifocal will be needed for close work.

For the best in outdoor seeing, you must provide all of the information you can about how you use your eyes. What is the toughest visual task? How long do you stay at it? How far away must you see things critically? Is there annoying glare? What kind of equipment do you use? Do not leave such questions unanswered. Above all, mention your outdoor avocation, even if you think it may not require special attention.

Quality of Lenses

If you must wear corrective lenses, they should be of the finest quality. Not all of them are. Just as scopes, binoculars, and cameras have lenses with optics of different quality, so do spectacle lenses. The clearness of the glass, its homogeneity, the smoothness of the surface polish, the absence of flaws of any kind are characteristics of top quality lenses. The opposite is frequently found in seconds, some imports, and a lot of inferior lenses.

Even though the glass itself may meet high optical standards, a lens must be designed properly to provide the best in seeing. This is especially important for the sportsman, who frequently gazes through all portions of a lens to inspect the outdoors. The movement of the eye takes the line of sight away from the optical center of the lens to its very edge.

Perfect focus is obtained only in the point known as the optical center of the lens. The explanation for this lies in the way the eye turns around a theoretical center of rotation, in the curvature of the retinal surface of the eye, and in certain optical principles which relate to the angles light rays make with curved surfaces. In stronger lens powers, the difference in focus from center to rim is significant, especially if the lens has not been designed to compensate for it.

Lenses made on "regular" base curves have considerable focus error away from the optical center. They are simpler and cheaper to make than lenses compensating for the error. Lenses called "corrected curve" lenses are generated on special base curves which minimize the focus difference from center to edge. Some reduce it almost completely. They are more difficult to manufacture therefore and cost more. In very high powers, even these lenses do not produce exactly the same focus at the edge as through the optical center.

Prismatic effects are created by all lenses, irrespective of their base curve, when the viewer is looking away from the optical center. This means images appear to be slightly displaced from their true direction. The amount of displacement depends upon the power of the lenses and the degree of eccentric fixation. If the power of one spectacle lens differs a great deal from the other, the prismatic effect can be important and the lens prescription should be compensated to make up for it. This is done by placement of optical centers, by putting prism in the lens, or more likely by modifying the lens power.

There is one situation in which the prismatic displacement of images through glasses might make a difference in the outdoors. That is when a gun is fired by a body-motor feeling of target direction alone—shooting skeet for example. In this case, the body muscle sense is directed by the eyes to judge that the target has a different position than it really has. Eyes see the target or bird slightly displaced because of the prisms but the body sense cannot correct for this since the gunsight is not seen visually. If the aim were by sight, the gunsight would be displaced by the same factor as the target and no error would result.

Quality of Multifocal Lenses

There is a great difference in quality of multifocal lenses. Some types of bifocals have advantages over others and these are described below. But in addition, any type of bifocal, for example, can be made very well or very badly. In bifocals two kinds of glass are used, each with a different index of refraction, one for the major lens and the other for the bifocal segment. In certain types of bifocals these two are fused by a heating process, and this is where things can go wrong.

Some bifocals create rainbow effects, distortion, and blur. Good lenses have coated edges on the segments themselves. Substandard lenses are not ground and polished to perfection. And of course, no matter what the lens quality, it should always be carefully checked to see that it is exactly the prescription that has been ordered.

Multifocal Lenses for Near Vision

Suppose you have reached the stage where extra lens power is necessary for close work. You may use "reading glasses" or bifocals, whichever fits your purpose better. (Reading glasses are any single vision lenses used for close seeing—reading, shop work, sighting a pistol—and they generally are too strong to see clearly at a distance.) You may give up to presbyopia reluctantly but when you do you must compensate for it in the most convenient way.

The weak focus has to be bolstered by extra lens power over and above any lens that may be required to correct distance vision. This is easy to provide, with an appropriate convex lens (a plus lens). But such a lens blurs distance vision since it focuses the eye for a near point. Rarely is it convenient for sports. The choice then is a multifocal lens. Bifocals have two areas of focus, one for distance seeing, one for near.

There are two variables involved in prescribing a bifocal to adapt it to exact needs.

1. The power of the bifocal segment can be selected for any distance desired. It could be made for seeing as close as eight to ten inches to tie a fly or do handwork on a gun stock. Or it could be set for twenty to thirty inches to see the dashboard of auto or airplane. But it probably cannot provide focus at both distances. The stronger the lens power, the smaller the in-and-out range it will provide. This linear range also depends upon how much focusing ability the eye itself still has.

2. The position of the bifocal segment and its size should be carefully determined. A bifocal is usually placed in the lower third of the lens but it need not be. It is only put there because most bifocals are made for working and reading, which are almost always performed in a centered and downward position. The bifocal can be at the top of the lens or in the corner, and it can be as small as a dime or encompass most of the lens.

Now if a multifocal lens is to be made in the proper combination of the variables of power and position, the person who writes the prescription must know exactly what the requirements are. This means you must be able to explain in detail what the near vision requirements are of your particular sport—whether details are critical, how long you stay at it, how far from your eyes the near vision point is and where it is in respect to your eyes (overhead, at eye level, off to one side).

Large bifocals have advantage for doing near work over a large area, as in a home workshop. In fact, the bifocal can be a bifield with the near-vision portion taking up the entire bottom half of the lens or more. The distance section can be only a small area at the top for looking up at a distance. But such a lens is highly vocational and would not likely be suitable for outdoor sports. In fact, few multi-

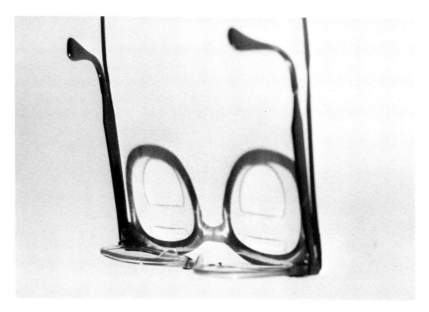

Double-segment bifocals are good for tasks requiring seeing up close and overhead.

focal lenses are the best for outdoors. The reason is that multifocals, having limited ranges of focus and usable near vision areas, must be tailored exactly to the individual's needs. And the demands of one job are far different from another. Studies have shown that only a few on-the-job multifocals are suitable for use by the sportsman.

A bifocal blurs the ground because it is focused closer than the ground distance. New bifocals are hardly advised for a hike over rough terrain. It may even be difficult to walk down your own driveway at first. The difficulty would be minimized if the bifocal were small and set low in the lens so it would be easy to look over it.

Small, low bifocals make walking easier but minimize the useful near vision area. For large ones, the opposite is true. Which kind should be used depends upon the goal. Sometimes medium-sized segments in a medium-high position are the best solution.

Get out the yardstick. Measure the exact distance from your eyes in normal position to where you must see. Indicate whether the seeing demand is primary (critical and intense), secondary, or gross. Specify where the location is with respect to eye level, and estimate in degree of angle if you can. With this information, you can obtain lenses to bring your vision back very near to its former efficiency.

What about bifocal shapes? The lens shape really depends upon what it is to be used for. Some of these points are covered in Part III, which deals with visual problems in specific sports and their solutions. A tiny round segment in the bottom of the lens is fine for golf, the pistol shooter can use a bifocal in the upper right-hand corner of the lens, while the fisherman may need a barrel-shaped segment which leaves a space beneath to see rocks as he wades into a stream.

Trifocals are unlikely to be suitable for sports, or outdoor use. The trifocal must set high in the lens and will produce ground blur. The person well adapted to it may get along but normally such a lens is not advised. On the other hand, the private pilot may like a trifocal for viewing instruments in the cockpit. The same is true of other highly vocational lenses; quadrifocals, inverted bifocals, or unusual placement of segments will not do for general outdoor sports but may be needed for specific tasks.

Bifocals are made in sunglass tints. The information in Chapter 9 about sunglasses applies equally to bifocals. Lighter tints are also available in pinks used indoors. The photochromic lens, which adapts from light to dark, is also made in a bifocal, although it limited to the one-piece type.

A one-piece bifocal is made of a single piece of glass, the different power in the bifocal segment being created by a differential grinding process. These segments are generally large and not really necessary for sport use; on the other hand, properly positioned ones may be acceptable. Most bifocals are fused from two pieces of glass, which can be made in almost any size and shape. Most lenses for use outdoors are fused bifocals. Multifocals can also be made in safety glass lenses and in plastic.

GETTING USED TO BIFOCALS

The two-focus lens does require an adjustment period. It is particularly annoying outdoors because of the need to look over the bifocal segment to see the ground clearly. Here are some tips about minimizing difficulties in wearing bifocals for sports.

1. Big jumps in lens power are hard to take; small ones are quite

easy. Thus, adjustments are much more rapid if bifocals are put on when first needed, and new prescriptions made as soon as vision changes sufficiently.

2. Be sure the bifocals are designed to exact needs, both in position in the lens and in power.

3. Learn the tricks of turning the eyes to look into the bifocal when near vision is needed. Tilt the head, get the bifocal out of the way to look at the ground. If they are done right from the first, proper head and eye movements soon become automatic.

4. Keep your glasses in perfect adjustment. To work the best, bifocals must be in precise alignment; even a slight variation in position can be the source of considerable annoyance.

5. Adjustment is faster if the bifocals are worn only for the purpose for which they were intended. You may need several pairs, in different powers and segment positions to provide the best vision for different requirements in outdoor sports.

OTHER SOLUTIONS TO NEAR-VISION PROBLEMS

There are two possible ways to avoid the bifocal problems. Both are a bit of nuisance but might be the choice of some individuals.

One is to use a separate pair of single vision lenses to see near objects. The person who requires a distance correction will then need two pairs of glasses. He can change from one to the other when necessary. Generally, a bifocal is a more convenient choice for the person who would need to change frequently.

Another method is to add lens power over the distance correction by a clip-on lens. This could even be a bifocal. It can be clipped onto glasses worn for distance or even onto sunlenses to provide near vision when needed. It can be removed of course when it is in the way.

The same result can be achieved by a flip-down lens. This is an arrangement like that used by the outfielder who flips down sunglasses when catching a fly in the sun. The frame can carry the distance correction, and the flip-down front can take a single vision reading lens or a bifocal into proper position.

Complex? Involved? A nuisance? Perhaps, but once the eye cannot adjust adequately by itself, there is no choice but one of the solutions suggested here. Sports are a lot easier if you select the one that fits you and your outdoor needs the best.

Lenses that Are Safe for Outdoor Use

The day will probably come when all glasses will have safety lenses. Several state laws require them now and the federal government is also considering such legislation. But the outdoorsman should not wait for laws to be enacted. Without safety lenses he faces considerable risk of eye injury, or at least broken lenses and the great inconvenience that can cause.

Naturally the hazards are greater for some sports than others. *Every* gunner should wear a safety lens whether he requires glasses otherwise or not. Though chance of permanent loss of sight is small, enough splatter and debris from ejected shells fill the area around a gunner's eyes to make seeing extremely hazardous. A tiny piece of dirt or metal embedded in the cornea can result in two weeks in the hospital, and blindness from it is possible. Even a slight injury will end the day's shooting and can be very painful. Such an incident can happen any time and with ordinary glass lenses can be most disastrous.

But even ordinary outdoor usage creates threats to eyesight. Limbs, leaves, dirt can flip in the eye when least expected. Dust and wind often fill eyes with tears. Scrambling through trees, tall weeds, and brush can cut, gouge, and bruise eyelids and eye tissue. What is needed is a protective shield. Safety lenses provide this very effectively if they are good lenses and large enough.

For industrial purposes, a glass safety lens is at least three millimeters thick and heat-treated so it will withstand the impact of a ⅞-inch steel ball dropped from a height of fifty inches. Such lenses are quite heavy and would be very bulky in large goggles. Outside of the rare possibility of a fractured breech, high velocity impact is not the outdoorsman's chief problem and a certain amount of breakage resistance might be sacrificed in favor of lighter weight and more comfort in outdoor glasses.

The three-millimeter industrial safety lens is called a *case-hardened* lens, or *industrial* lens. Such terms as *impact-resistant, tempross, junior hardened, safety hardened,* and *tempered* generally refer to lenses which are heat-treated but do not have the industrial thickness. Such lenses are at least two millimeters thick and of course heat-treated. They will withstand the impact of a ⅝-inch steel bar dropped from fifty inches. These lenses are only a little thicker than ordinary lenses.

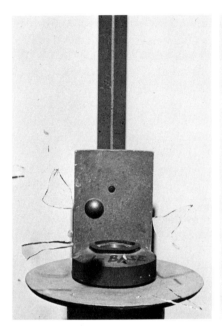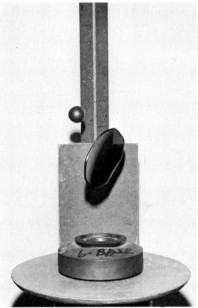

The drop ball test is used to check safety lenses. The lens on the left is ordinary glass, easily shattered by the steel ball dropped from a height of one meter. The heat-treated lens on the right, which is a sunlens designed for sportsmen, does not break from the impact. *(Courtesy of Bausch & Lomb)*

In fact, few lenses are made thinner than two millimeters in the thinnest spot. Break-resistant lenses of this type usually look no different from regular lenses. But any lens—any multifocal, any tint—is safe *only* if it is thick enough and heat-treated.

Heat-treated glass can be broken. But it tends to crumble into fragments rather than into the sharp-edged splinters which are so dangerous. Also safety lenses are less likely to break under the rough handling they so often get outdoors. For that reason alone, they are wise economy.

The so-called "safe" shooting lens is at least two millimeters thick, sometimes a little more, but there is no guarantee of this. Today all shooting lenses produced by reputable firms are impact resistant. This is probably adequate for ordinary shooting and to protect against foreign objects when hunting, but they are not as strong as case-hardened lenses.

Many of the ordinary sunglasses on the market today are also made with safe lenses. These are the ones made by the best manufacturers, but they are not always labeled as being safe lenses. Be sure to ask about this and do not use sunglasses that are not safe if you face any risks of eye injury.

How can you tell if a lens is safe? Lenses can be checked on a Colmascope, a device for polarizing light which will show the strain pattern created by the heating process. Follow professional advice in the selection of safe outdoor glasses. If you have prescription lenses, the heat treating was done in the laboratory and checked before delivery to you. But if you are not sure of other glasses, have them checked by the polarized light test.

The hardening process realigns an outer envelope of molecules in the lens into a stronger form. This is how the polarizing test works, it reveals the "strain" pattern of molecular tension. This is also why a lens becomes unsafe if it is pitted or scratched. Any upset in the molecular structure, such as is caused by a nick in the surface, weakens the lens. Handle your safety glasses carefully, inspect them for breaks in the surface. Old lenses may give you a sense of false security and actually offer no real protection.

Plastic Lenses

What about plastic for safety? Cuts and scratches hardly matter; plastic has good safety qualities, and it can be made into prescription lenses including bifocals. There are several drawbacks to even the best optical plastic however. It scratches more easily than glass so must be handled rather carefully, and there is a limitation in the absorption properties of tinted plastic lenses.

Plastic lenses, though unbreakable, are normal in appearance. They are particularly useful in eye-hazardous occupations since they are more resistant to high-speed impact than other types of safety glasses. They do not need to be made extra thick to be safe.

With their weight less than half that of ordinary glass lenses, plastic offers maximum wearing comfort. Weight is a problem for many people requiring "strong" glass lenses. The tension and pressure on nose and ears can be reduced by plastic lenses. The cost is greater

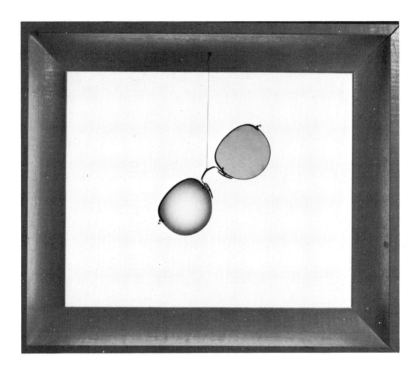

The right lens, of tinted plastic, shows uniformity of light distribution. The left lens is glass in the same prescription; it demonstrates not only greater weight but uneven light absorption. *(Courtesy of Armorlite, Inc.)*

than for glass lenses but safety and weight advantages may well be worth the extra expense. Plastic is being more widely used for prescription lenses. Almost all opthalmic lenses are made from a plastic base known as CR-39, a thermosetting allyl-diglycol-carbonate.

The best optical plastic is crystal clear, relatively free from imperfections, and offers excellent vision. It must be manufactured very carefully. The lenses are fog-resistant; they do not collect moisture nor "smear up" as easily as ordinary glasses. This is another advantage for outdoor use.

However, plastic lenses do present a problem. Since the material is not rigid like glass, pressure exerted against the edges can cause it to bulge and distort slightly. This can happen when the lens fits too tightly in the frame, and the result is a change in the prescription, which will affect seeing. The problem is not easy to detect with the devices used to check lens power. If you have plastic lenses which are the right prescription but are uncomfortable, have them inspected to be sure the frame edge is not putting pressure on the lens and causing distortion.

Plastic lenses can be dyed any color. Many of the tints used in plastic lenses are too light for outdoor use and are purely cosmetic. Even in dark greys and acceptable tints, there may be fading since the dyes plastic will absorb are not stable. If you have plastic lenses, check them from time to time to see if they are holding their color.

Lens Coating

Ghost images and annoying reflections are seen by many spectacle wearers. These spots and shadows are often so troublesome as to make a fine prescription useless. Yet they can be very easily eliminated by properly coating the lenses.

Each of the two surfaces of a spectacle lens acts as a little mirror. It reflects lights and objects, even the image of one's eye can be seen wearing some glasses. This scattered light reduces visibility and can produce considerable discomfort. It produces the same effect as blurred and fuzzy vision, particularly outdoors or at night.

Treatment of ophthalmic lenses with a metallic coating process gets rid of the ghost images and makes vision clearer. "Coating" is commonplace on camera lenses, binoculars, and most optical instruments. The same process can be effectively used on spectacle lenses to improve their light transmission.

The coating is a layer of metal, four millionths of an inch thick, which fuses with the glass. Its anti-reflection properties serve to cut out the stray light and allow more light to pass through the lens to become useful to seeing. There are various kinds of coatings but they all accomplish about the same goals.

Coatings can be added in various densities and colors. Since they are put on the surface of the lenses, it is possible to take a pair of spectacle—a second pair, for example—and by adding a heavy coating of the desired tint, make them into sunglasses. By selection of proper coating material, the light transmission properties of a lens can be carefully controlled.

Coating is especially useful for outdoor use. Even sunglasses can

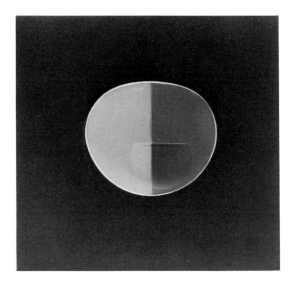

The right half of this lens is coated. The left half is not and reflects so much bright photographic light that the uncoated side appears almost grey. *(Courtesy of Pacific Universal Products Corporation)*

be coated to reduce reflections from the lens surfaces. The veiling glare from the lenses themselves can reduce imagery a good deal. Some kinds of prescriptions create more reflections than others. At night, bright reflection of lights can also be minimized.

One type of coating is reflective. It is practically colorless and reduces light reflections at the two lens surfaces by enabling the light to pass through without being reflected. This actually increases the amount of light which will pass through by as much as 6 percent. Though not a great boost, it is somewhat helpful in seeing dim objects at night. Dense reflective coatings can reflect a great deal of light and have a "mirror" look to them.

Absorptive coatings can also be used. They absorb certain wave lengths and therefore appear colored, the color of the wavelengths not absorbed. If it is not too restrictive in the wavelengths absorbed, such a coating can make a good sunglass for outdoors.

Very light absorptive coatings—the fad tints of pastels from purple to chartreuse—are for glamour only. They are solely fashion items and in narrow spectrum colors have no place outdoors. They may not hinder seeing as long as they do not cut down the light significantly or create color perception variation. On the other hand, they should not be relied on to protect against high glare.

Getting Used to Glasses

A well-known complaint is that new glasses are "hard to get used to." But many troubles are more imaginary than real. Alarmed by the visual distortion or the downright discomfort created by first spectacles, or a change in old ones, some people use them only half-heartedly. This prolongs the adjustment period. As a result, even after a long time, adaptation may not be complete. Half the battle in getting used to glasses is knowing what to expect.

Typical effects during the period of adjustment to glasses are: ground appears to slant, walls tilt, objects look too big or too small, things "swim" around, or reading may seem difficult. Even blur, headache, or dizziness may develop at first. These sensations can be explained by the optical effects produced by certain types of lenses. The severity of the distortions depends not only upon the exact nature of the lens prescription, but also upon individual sensitivity and adaptability.

The "getting used to glasses period" is ordinarily a matter of a week to a month. After a few days, the symptoms should begin to disappear. In a week, the effects may be noticeable only briefly or under certain conditions; while at the end of a month the process is generally complete. New lenses may bother a person at one time and not another. His emotional state, health, and understanding of the problem all play a part. These may lengthen the adjustment time to months or in a rare case, even longer.

Here are some ways to speed up getting used to glasses:

1. *Be sure to understand the instructions about the use of your glasses and follow them exactly.* Discuss the matter with your optometrist thoroughly and find out what your glasses will and will not do. Do not expect the impossible.

2. *Wear the lenses first in familiar surroundings and for easy jobs.* You will probably have less trouble indoors; distortions in your space world will be worse when walking outside.

3. *Forget your new glasses, don't fight them.* Your problem may be imaginary, or at least magnified, if you "experiment" with your

spectacles or are too conscious of them. Look *through* your glasses, not *at* them.

4. *Depending upon professional advice, take some rest periods without your glasses, or wear your old ones now and then.* When you break in new shoes, it is generally better to walk around the block the first day than to take a ten-mile hike.

5. *Once the adaptation has well begun, wear your glasses regularly.* You cannot get used to glasses which are lying in the dresser drawer. Use them as you have been instructed if you really want to get the most from your eyes.

There are references in this book to vocational lenses. In a sense, all lens prescriptions are vocational—that is, they are designed to meet certain special needs. They work best in solving certain seeing problems—firing a gun, or playing golf, or skin diving, or doing camp chores. They may not work as well for doing other things.

To adjust easily and to get the best results from glasses especially designed for your sporting needs, you should use them solely for those needs. Lenses with a tiny bifocal to make walking around in the mountains easy will not work well at a desk. Wear glasses for the purpose for which they were designed. And generally you'll get far better performance if they are especially designed for whatever your outdoor sport.

chapter **7**

all about

frames

To tell literally *all* about frames is more than necessary. This chapter will tell you *enough* about frames to guide you in selecting eyewear for your outdoor needs. And certainly frames are vital to your comfort and good seeing.

Long ago man struggled with many kinds of materials to create a frame that was comfortable and serviceable. They were made of bone, leather, cloth, rubber, wood, tortoise shell, and metal. He worked harder at producing a frame that rested comfortably on his nose and ears than he did at making lenses.

Ingenious devices were invented to keep the frames on. Some had bands that went around the head, others sported strings that tied on the ears or pins that fastened them to the hat—the latter, it was said, were "only good for princes who didn't have to give a salute." The earpieces, or *temples* as they are correctly called, were made in practically every way man could devise. Some were flexible, some were stiff and fitted the head in a clamp-like action, some were adjustable to take up the slack. Many were wrapped and covered at the tips to prevent cutting the ears.

Developing a comfortable bridge challenged man's ingenuity. Some bridges were adjustable, others pinched the nose and made welts. There were rigid bars, spring devices, contour shapes and "floating" pads. The pads were made of rubber, wood, shell, and sponge. In the late nineteenth century, hundreds and hundreds of patents were granted for frames with many variations of bridges, temples, hinges, and design.

The sportsman was not left out. Goggles were devised for driving in the early open touring cars. The frames were large and close fitting, even having side shields to keep out wind and dust. Some had cloth or wool around the rims so the entire frame edge could fit tightly against the face.

One of the most unique frames ever devised had an extremely practical purpose. The inventor, H. Gifford, describes the frame in his own words:

Having been much annoyed while playing tennis or doing any hard work in hot weather by sweat running down from my eyebrows upon my glasses, I have had a pair of gutters made in aluminum which screw onto the sides of the bridge and the outside posts which prevent this trouble. The inner edge of the gutter fits close under the eyebrows and carries any excessive perspiration off to the sides. I think the frame may find a larger application among farmers than among tennis players, as any one who has attempted to pitch hay or do other hard work in the hot sun will readily appreciate. Many a farmer who ought to wear glasses either for visual purposes or to protect his only remaining eye will not do so on account of the dimming of the glasses in hot weather.

The frames of even a few years ago are a far cry from those used today. Frames now are not only much more comfortable than in the past but are made better. The strong style factor has, however, tended to minimize some of the optical qualities of frames with regard to size, shape, and position of the lens with respect to the eye.

What kinds of frames are best? There is no easy answer. Quality metal or plastic are both good for spectacle frames, but many grades and types of metal and plastic are used in manufacture.

Plastic Frames

Plastic makes excellent frames providing strength and comfort. Two kinds are used. Most early plastic frames were cellulose nitrate (celluloid). It had a few advantages for frames but two big disadvantages that have practically eliminated it in American manufacture. However it is still used in other countries.

Cellulose nitrate is highly inflammable. It has been to known to catch fire while being worn, so the wearer is obliged to handle such glasses with special care and take fire precautions. But celluloid frames are still on the market in the form of cheap imports, and certain frames brought in by tourists may be of this inflammable material.

The other disadvantage of cellulose nitrate is that it will not hold color very well. An attractive pink frame will slowly turn yellow, especially if worn much outdoors. Delicate colors are hard to produce and hold. There may still be a few cellulose nitrate frames around. One way to tell is to heat them slightly (be careful); if they are nitrate they will give off a camphor smell. Several state legislatures have considered bills to outlaw such frames.

Cellulose acetate has replaced the nitrate frame. It is noninflammable and holds color quite well. This is obviously the best kind of frame for outdoor use. This recommendation also applies to plastic shields, goggles, and helmets.

Plastics used in frames are thermoplastics, which means that they can be hardened by cooling but will soften when reheated. Such a characteristic is essential in order to insert the lens and make adjustments. Good plastic frames also have "memory"—after being stretched, they will return to their original size and shape. Poor frames will not. (Plastic lenses inside the frame are made of thermosetting material. Once this kind of plastic has hardened by a heating process, it does not soften again.)

Cheap plastic frames can look stylish but are seldom durable. Look carefully at the finish of the plastic to see if it is smooth, uniform, and neatly finished. Inspect the hinges; they should be made of strong metal and be well-machined. Compare the workmanship on a fine prescription frame with the dime store variety and you will find a big difference.

The plastic temples on most good frames have a wire core to

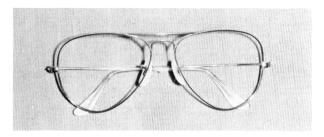

An excellent frame for outdoor wear. This one is sturdy and well made, with face-form contour in a large size. It is also available with temples that wrap around the ears.

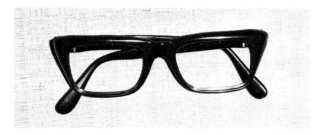

A nylon frame is tough and flexible, also lightweight. This shape is good; such a frame must fit perfectly on the bridge.

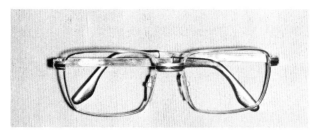

All-metal frame with an adjustable pad bridge, designed for style. Be sure of quality of metal in such frames; not all are gold-filled material.

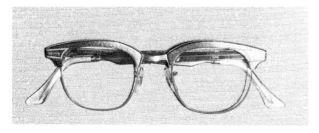

A very serviceable frame with aluminum top rim and temples; lens rim is top quality metal. Size might be a limitation for outdoor use if broad coverage is needed.

make them stronger. Look for this. It may be hidden under the dark plastic but be sure it is there. The wire core also keeps the temples stiff and in better adjustment.

Frames with metal braced fronts are also made. Manufacturers have long made them available for youngsters since the rough and tumble set snap plastic frame fronts as if it were a game. For some reason, there has been a reluctance to make these frames which stand up better available to adults, but at least one manufacturer produces braced-front frames in a full range of sizes for adults.

Nylon Frames

Nylon is also used to make frames. It is much more flexible than plastic and will not break so easily. It is lightweight and durable. It is not very popular because it cannot be made in the great variety of colors with mottled effects. For outdoor use, however, it is very satisfactory.

For comfort, the plastic or nylon frame rates high. This is because of the kind of bridge it has—a wide plastic band resting on a portion of the bridge of the nose. Shapes can be either the saddle or the keyhole. One fits some people better than the other. But the plastic bridge is the most comfortable bridge for the most people.

Metal Frames

A number of kinds of metal have been used for frames. The top of the line is a gold-filled material, usually 1/10 of twelve karats. It is widely used for spectacle frames, has style and durability, and can easily be adjusted. It is used for the best quality goggles, for plastic-metal combination frames, and for most rimless glasses. Ask what metal is used in the production of any frame you are considering.

Other metal is used to imitate the effect of gold or silver frames. Careful inspection easily reveals the difference. For one thing, the 1/10 of twelve karat material always has that designation engraved on the frame; it is small and hard to find but it is always there. Nickel silver is used in frames for industrial safety lenses. They are good frames but one finds all sorts of inferior metal used in others.

Inferior metal frames are soft and bend, even break, very easily. Some are affected by the acidity of the skin and must be covered with plastic to prevent corrosion. The worst problem develops in trying to adjust these frames. If not too soft, they often are too brittle, and so they cannot be bent to let the pads fit comfortably on the wearer's nose. The parts are usually not replaceable.

Frames are like so many other materials—the less they cost, the poorer their quality, and the less service they give. There are a few exceptions, but generally good frames cost more and are worth it.

Examine a metal frame carefully. Notice how it is machined. Check the hinges and rivets. Inspect the finish to see if it is smooth and regular. Thickness is not especially important, so frames need not be heavy. Be sure the temples used fit the frame front very well.

Aluminum alloys are now widely used in farmes. Some solid rim frames are produced of aluminum. They must be rather thick to resist bending easily, or have a bridge of stiffer metal. These types are like all-plastic frames with saddle or keyhole bridges. They have been widely used in women's frames but not very popular for men —perhaps because they appear heavy and bulky in the large sizes used by men.

Metal frames, the gold-filled type especially, are excellent for outdoor use. They are strong and give the lens edge good protection without requiring a heavy rim, which not only restricts the view somewhat but also gets in the way of some wearers.

Except for the all-aluminum ones, most metal frames have adjustable rocking pads. These are both an asset and a liability. They are quite adjustable so the frame can be raised or lowered, or set close to or farther from the face. With a plastic frame, the amount of adjustment possible is very limited, though there is a little.

The adjustability plus the good field of view without the heavy frame edge, gives the metal frame some optical advantages. Its big drawback is the bridge. All the frame and lens weight rests on the small pads fitted to the side of the bridge of the nose. This does not bother some people but others cannot stand it. Such a bridge has to be fitted very carefully to the individual.

The rocking pad bridge is cooler, a considerable advantage outdoors. The metal frame sets away from the face slightly while the plastic one, being closer, traps heat behind it. To what degree also depends upon the wearer's physical features. But for active sports, the free-standing frame lessens the moisture on the lenses—or the need for the frame with downspouts like the invention of Gifford.

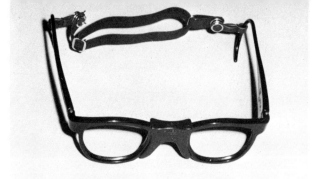

Athletic frames like this with lenses of plastic or hardened glass can be worn in contact sports. Rubber bridge protects nose from a blow.

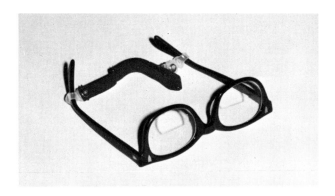

Elastic band can be attached to any pair of glasses.

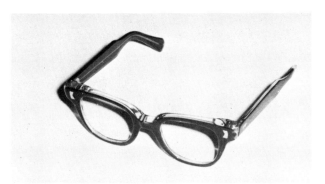

Heavy-weight plastic frame, rugged for outdoor use.

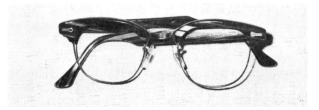

A combination metal and plastic frame, very adjustable for good fit.

Rimless Eyeglasses

For safety reasons and to avoid the risk of breakage, rimless glasses are hardly recommended for outdoors unless they have plastic lenses. Lenses must be drilled for mounting in rimless frames, but the molecular structure of a glass safety lens will not form the protective envelope properly if it is disturbed by holes. Actually the drilling is done first, then the lens heat-treated, but such a lens is not safe. So never have glass safety lenses put in a rimless frame. The plastic lens, however, is safe even if drilled and mounted in a rimless frame.

Rimless frames have all of the advantages of adjustability, good visibility, lightness, and comfort. With plastic lenses, they can be the most comfortable spectacles possible. Their one drawback is that they do get out of adjustment rather easily and this might make them unsuitable for some outdoor sports.

This book is not considering style in frames. These will change. Granny styles are here today and will be gone tomorrow. But the fundamentals of good fit and function will not change. A sturdy, adjustable frame, with maximum visibility and plenty of comfort will always be the best bet for sport. If such a frame is also in style, fine, but do not select frames for looks alone if you want the best for outdoor use.

Special Frames

There are some special kinds of frames made for use in heavy action. Elastic bands are also available to be attached to any kind of spectacle frame. They attach to the temple ends and go behind the head, and the tension can be adjusted. A special athletic frame is made with a soft rubber bridge. It is of very durable metal and has temples that wrap snugly around the ears. With safety glass lenses or plastic, it can be worn for contact sports.

Frame Sizes

Prescription frames come in a number of sizes with three elements to consider which vary in size independently of each other.

Bridges are made in as many as four or five sizes which differ in width in two millimeter steps. In a few instances, larger ones are available on special order, but getting them often takes an impractically long time.

Do not judge the feel of a frame from a sample. For one thing, it probably has no lenses in it and these will add half the total weight. Let the fitter pick the right bridge and temple dimension for you and adjust the frame to comfort. However, you may want to have something to say about how large a lens size should be—only you can determine if a small size would annoy you because you are conscious of seeing the frame edge.

Frames come in as many as seven or eight (most of them fewer) lens sizes. They differ also in two millimeter steps, which may not seem like much but can make a big difference when worn. For outdoor use, get as large a size as needed to fill your field of view—not saucers of course, nor something so outlandish in size that they look terrible. Remember that face-form shapes are the best, especially for sunglasses. Get the frame edge out of the way for the most natural kind of seeing without a fenced-in feeling.

The temples are measured in inches. Though several other sizes are needed for youngsters, nearly all adults are fitted with temples from 5¼ to 6¾ inches long. A quarter inch in temple length can make the difference between comfort and security and a pair slipping off to the bottom of the lake. Too long is as bad as too short. There is only one length temple to get—one that is just right for you, and this decision should be left up to professional advice. Point out that you wear glasses in sports and that they must fit snugly in place. Consider the wrap-around temple (which wraps around the ear rather than folding over part of the way behind the ear and pressing against the head) with flexible metal tips. They hold on better than any other type.

Keeping Frames in Adjustment

All sorts of ingenious devices have been developed to make frames more comfortable and stay in place. Rubber galoshes can be put over rocking pads on metal frames, plastic temple covers exist in half a dozen styles, rubber bands can be put over hinges to give spring to the temples, and stay-on tips added to keep temples behind the ears. The best solution is the right frame in the first place.

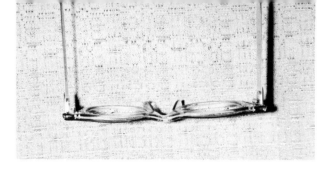

Plastic frame with metal-braced front. A band of metal runs across the top inside the plastic to strengthen the bridge, where breakage is most likely to occur.

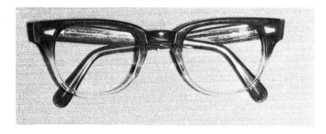

Plastic frame with clear bottom edges which do not interfere with vision in a downward direction.

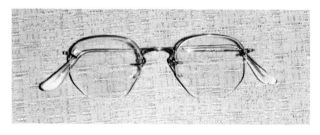

Rimless frame, lightweight and very comfortable. Safest for outdoor wear with plastic lenses.

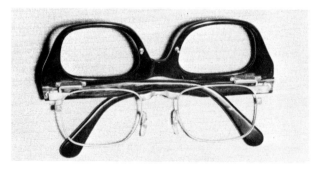

Metal frame with flip-down plastic front. In this way a sunlens or extra lens power can be flipped down in front of the eyes when needed.

But if your frame just refuses to fit right or stay in place, try some of the improvisations, at least temporarily.

Which stays up better, the bridge with the rocking pads that pinch the nose or the plastic saddle bridge? If glasses slide down, the bridge is not at fault. Too wide or too narrow a bridge will make the frames set low or high but only the temples hold the frame up.

Keep your frames in perfect adjustment. Comfort is reason enough, convenience is another. Frames that hurt will end up in the pocket. So will ones you have to hold on with one hand while trying to line up a putt. But unless you are particularly careful in handling your spectacles or have them adjusted to fit your face and eye position, you may be getting far less vision than you should.

The effectiveness of some lenses can be altered as much as 50 percent by ill-fitting, twisted frames. The power of a pair of spectacle lenses is correct only if they are positioned exactly thirteen millimeters in front of the eye. Optical lenses have a center which must be precisely placed. All glasses are designed to set at a certain angle on the face, and any variation from these positions will prevent the wearer from getting the focus which was ordered for him.

The stronger the lens, the more critical its adjustment. Some eyes are more sensitive to lens positions than others. Bifocals and trifocals require exacting alignment regardless of their strength. They must also be centered for the distance between the eyes. Bifocals should be level and not too high, especially for wear outdoors.

Head and neck posture are affected if glasses get out of line. Once a person is accustomed to glasses in a certain position, he will experience considerable discomfort and annoyance from any change. Blur and eyestrain of an indefinite sort may be the clue to the need for adjustment of the glasses.

Visual efficiency is sure to suffer if glasses are not kept in exact position. In addition, the frame itself can be troublesome, though it may not directly affect eyesight. Pressure of the frame on nose and ears can create tension and headache, and sometimes eyes get the blame. Skin irritations and annoying sore spots can be created if frames do not set properly. Individual tolerance to lens adjustment varies a great deal, but all glasses should be adjusted periodically.

chapter **8**

contact lenses

Some of the seeing problems discussed in previous chapters would be eliminated if the outdoorsman wore contact lenses. Others would be created, however; so the pros and cons of contacts should be weighed very carefully before deciding they are the best for outdoor sports.

For people with relatively mild visual problems, contacts are generally not worth the time and trouble. This is an individual matter of course and depends upon how a person evaluates "time and trouble." But contacts may have a lot to offer to people with large visual errors.

Generally it is not satisfactory to wear contact lenses for sport alone. A few athletes in active sports like football and basketball can do this but only because of the brief period of a game. During these periods of high emotional stress and extreme physical activity, contacts are tolerable; in a less stressful situation, they would not be. The problem is that the eye does not adapt well to contacts with very limited wearing. Contact lens experts recommend that lenses be worn most of the time in order for the eyes to maintain good adaptation. Part-time wear does not work well and the wearer seldom attains maximum comfort.

In rough sports, exertion and impact can knock the lenses out of the eyes, or at least displace them from their normal position on the cornea. This can happen when the lids blink hard during sudden physical activity or to duck a coming blow or upset. But otherwise contact lenses present no particular difficulties for sport and outdoor wear.

People who are not completely dependent upon glasses generally should not wear contact lenses. If glasses are not required all of the time, even though they are necessary for outdoor sports, contacts may not be worth the bother. The sportsman must weigh the inconvenience of contacts against the nuisances of spectacle frames and lenses.

Frames are hot, can be uncomfortable on the face, slide down, require constant adjustment, wear out, break easily, restrict the field of view, change style, and are a bother to pack, handle, and remember to take on an outing. On the other hand, they are easy to put on and take off, hold lenses very efficiently, are relatively inexpensive, can be repaired, improve the looks of some people, and carry multifocal lenses very well.

Lenses break unless given special treatment or are made of plastic, they scratch from careless handling, are perfect only at the optical center, must be of good quality to produce the exact prescription near the lens edge, limit the field of view and require frequent changing to keep up with variations in the state of refraction of the eye. But they do produce good seeing, are easy to get used to, cost relatively little, can be made in a great variety of multifocals, and are easily available in several different prescriptions for various uses.

Contact lenses require considerable time for adaptation, are expensive to fit, are small and difficult to handle, and can be lost quite easily. They cannot be worn all day by some people, they require careful cleaning and care each day, may not completely do away with the need for eyeglasses, are not entirely satisfactory in multifocals, and cannot be changed easily to go from one prescription to another. Periodic inspection of the eyes wearing contacts is essential.

The advantages of contacts are many: they free the wearer from frames and lenses; vision through them (depending upon the individual case) is generally excellent; there are no problems of optical centers, since the lens moves with the eye; peripheral vision is good; they generally do not have to be changed as frequently as spectacle lenses; there is no reflection, as with glass lenses, and no risk of breakage; and the mechanical problems of frame adjustments are eliminated.

How these factors of spectacles versus contacts are evaluated depends upon the individual. Looks are a big factor too, of course. There is no doubt that vanity is one of the most common reasons people decide on contacts. So the person who is absolutely dependent upon glasses, who detests frames and the restricted field of view they create, and who particularly thinks he or she looks better not wearing spectacles will probably do well in contact lenses. If none of these facts apply, chances of success are rather slim.

There are exceptions. A few people who have only mild prescriptions and need lenses only occasionally, do get along reasonably well with contacts. They however are strongly motivated. Motivation is really the key to success.

Occasionally physical and physiological reasons prevent a person from wearing contacts with comfort. These relate to curvature of the cornea, the strength of the lids, the blinking reflex, and the tear fluid production system which keeps the eye moist. There is also a sensitivity factor, some eyes are more delicate than others. But only a few people cannot be fitted with contacts for any of these reasons.

Assuming that after a realistic look at the advantages and disadvantages of contact lenses for general use, the balance of the arguments is in favor of them. The motivation factor exists and there are no anatomical or optometric reasons for not wearing them. What about using contact lenses in the outdoors?

On the basis of the good vision they produce in many cases, contact lenses have the edge over eyeglasses. As mentioned above, the tiny piece of plastic rests neatly on the cornea and moves as the eye moves. Thus, the line of sight is always at, or near, the center of the lens. There is some lag of the lens as the eye moves, depending upon how tightly the lens is fitted. But the problems of looking through the lens edge of spectacles are eliminated and the hunter or marksman can see well no matter how he aims.

Fitting over the cornea as it does, the contact lens can in some cases provide better visual acuity than ordinary lenses. It replaces the cornea as a refracting surface and can compensate for some of its irregularities possible no other way. Therefore, some eyes get better vision with contacts.

But some eyes do not achieve as good visual acuity with contacts. This happens when there is some residual astigmatism produced by the crystalline lens of the eye. Special types of contact lenses can be ground to correct this but there is the possibility that acuity with contacts will not be maximum.

Visual acuity is an expression of the greatest resolving power the eye can produce—20/20 or whatever. This is a measure of central vision and of course it is a very important measure. But a person with only 20/30 vision with contacts will often maintain that he sees better than he did with spectacles which produced 20/20. What he means is that his "overall" seeing is better. He sees better because there is no restriction of the field by lenses and frames. Besides that, in every direction of gaze with contacts he has the maximum acuity, 20/30 in this example. With spectacles visual acuity in many areas may fall below that when he is forced to look through lens edges.

Probably the greatest value of contact lenses for sport is the clear overall field of view. Elimination of the physical problems of frames —the slipping and sliding, the heaviness and annoyance—would rank second. Eyes are safer with contact lenses too since there is no glass in front of the eye.

All is not on the plus side, however. Even if there are no problems of wearing the lenses—they fit comfortably and vision is good —the outdoor environment can cause some difficulties. Sun and dust are the main culprits. Humidity, altitude, and temperature have also been proposed as factors affecting the wear-ability of contacts, but scientific studies have yet to prove any such relationship. Contact lenses have been worn successfully in arctic regions, in the desert, by mountain climbers, and sky divers. However, wearing contacts in water, especially salt water, has been found annoying to some.

Excessive sun is troublesome to some contact lens wearers. This is because sensitivity to glare is increased—an especially frequent occurrence among beginning wearers. Sunglasses with no-focus lenses often need to be worn over contacts, thereby negating some of their advantages, since frames are again perched on the nose and lenses parked in front of the eye.

Another solution is contact lenses with a sunglass tint. These can be made in any tint desired. Since contact lenses are plastic, they can be dyed in the same way plastic spectacle lenses are. The only

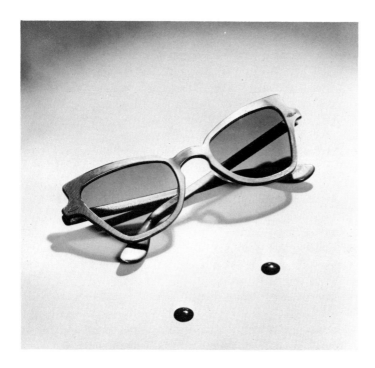

Size comparison of tinted contact lenses and ordinary sunglasses. *(Courtesy of the National Eye Research Foundation)*

drawback to sunglass lenses is the time and caution needed to change from clear to dark ones and back to clear—obviously more of a problem than putting on or taking off a pair of sunglasses.

A very real deterrent to wearing contact lenses outdoors is the possibility of dust getting behind the lenses. A speck of dirt feels like a boulder when trapped between a contact lens and the cornea. It can create a violent reaction of the eyelids, which close down hard and make it difficult to remove the lens. Such an experience can be disastrous for an inexperienced wearer and it is certainly no fun for an oldtimer. In extremely dusty conditions it may be impossible to wear contacts.

The reason some wearers report they do fine with contacts in some environments and poorly in others may be due to allergies rather than heat, temperature, and humidity. A person getting lenses for outdoor sports should discuss the purposes for which he will use the lens with the specialist who fits him. The question of allergies should be considered, even if he has not been subject to them otherwise.

Sometimes fitting methods for outdoor wear are different than for general use. For example, professional football players are often fitted with contact lenses that are very large and rest on the sclera (the white part of the eyeball). They are less likely to be dislodged by a flying tackle. Even with lenses resting entirely on the cornea, as most of them do, the larger the lens, the tighter it fits, and the less likely it is to be knocked off.

Not all eyes can be fitted with tight lenses. If you want to wear contacts for certain sports, the determining factor may be how tight a lens your eye will tolerate. Or if it is important enough to you, a larger and tighter pair of lenses may be necessary for outdoor use than you wear regularly.

The kind of lenses used, whether large or small, depends upon many factors that relate to the physical characteristics of the eyeball and the eyelids. Some lenses have small openings to permit fluid to pass through, some have weight at the bottom to hold them in place, some are curved more, some less than the surface of the eye itself. But none of these variables relate to wearing lenses outdoors. With the outdoor lens as with the indoor lens, good fit is what counts.

Multifocals in contact lenses are much more difficult to use than single vision lenses. There are optical and anatomical reasons why the lens must be positioned exactly right with respect to the lower lid. For the casual near seeing needs of some outdoor sports, bifocal contact lenses might be satisfactory. But most people find it necessary to wear eyeglasses over contacts in order to see close objects well.

chapter **9**

what you should
know about
sunglasses

Every year sportsmen spend millions of dollars on sunglasses with little or no knowledge of what they are getting. The result is a nationwide headache, lots of eyestrain, hazardous seeing, and wasted dollars.

The rush to get relief from the glare of the sun is not new. The Chinese wore tinted lenses fourteen centuries ago, long before corrective spectacles were invented. Eskimos and Himalayans utilized glare-protective devices for many years, and man has worn a hat to shade his eyes almost since the beginning of time. This suggests that the human eye never could operate with maximum comfort in the overbrightness outdoors.

Today the need for eye relief is great. Man has kicked up volumes of dust and poured tons of debris into the air. This atmospheric haze scatters light, makes glare more aggravating. (Perhaps you have noticed less need for sunglasses on a clear day than on a hazy one.) But whatever your reasons for wearing sunglasses—inherent nature of your eyes, habit patterns, or just the desire to be in style—if you feel better and see better in them, wear them. They offer many advantages, provided they are of good quality.

Value of Wearing Sunglasses

Squinting in the sun can build up fatigue. The price is discomfort, slowing down, loss of ability to perform. You also risk accident and injury if your visual performance is below par. And sunglasses are important whether mountain climbing or relaxing in camp.

A hat will reduce the overhead brightness and make vision more comfortable. Naturally it must have a broad brim to be effective. There is no doubt that the hat cuts total light entering the eye. But light can still be reflected into the eye from the ground surface. Sand, snow, water, and pavement reflect a great deal. Playground, greens, tundra, any heavy groundcover are less reflective.

Some studies suggest that reflected light is more annoying than direct light. Such light is scattered and diffuse. Sunglasses will block this, and polarizing filters will cut reflections and get rid of veiling glare.

Though reducing amount of light is their chief value, sunglasses have assets you might never guess. The best glasses filter out harmful rays which can damage the tissues of the eye. Many sportsmen have heard of "snow blindness," an extremely distressing condition caused by excessive radiation. However, even considerably lesser degrees of exposure can produce irritations, although they are milder.

Some experts believe that cataracts develop in the lens of the eye if it receives too much of certain rays. This does not mean that wearing sunglasses will insure that you never develop a cataract, or that cataracts are certain to develop if you do not. But the ideal sunlens should absorb wavelengths that have potentially dangerous properties. Certainly these rays are not useful in seeing.

The harmful rays are ultraviolet and infrared. The amounts of each in sunlight vary with geography, altitude, and season. Eye damage from them also depends upon intensity and length of exposure. The twice-a-year fisherman is in little danger, while the guide who is out nearly every day could conceivably be affected if he neglects to wear absorptive lenses.

Wearing sunglasses in the bright sun will help you see better at night, as was pointed out in Chapter 4. The rate and level of dark

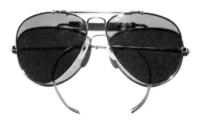

Sunglasses for sports featuring grey lenses, face-form shape; these give good coverage and the metal frame provides a good fit.

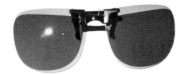

Polarizing plastic fitover; this one is lightweight and can easily be flipped up out of the way.

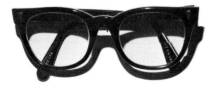

Photochromic bifocal lenses which darken as light increases.

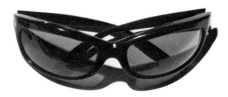

Wrap-around styles are good if not too narrow and if lenses are not so curved as to create distortion near the edges.

adaptation is increased if the visual cells are protected from too much visible light. When very dark lenses are used, the improvement may be as much as tenfold.

For driving on well-lighted streets, the gain in night vision produced by using sunglasses during the day is not highly significant. However, for flying a plane or piloting a boat at night, hiking or fishing in the dark, even working around camp, it can be meaningful.

Take sunglasses off at dusk. *Never* wear them at night. No tinted lens helps night vision, even for driving; it actually reduces the amount of available light. Neither should sunglasses be worn indoors even in the finest artificial illumination.

The disadvantages of sunglasses hardly count in normal activities. Care and handling are a bit of a nuisance. So is feel of the frame on the face. Cost and upkeep are nothing compared to benefits. Sunglasses are not habit forming—you may become "dependent" upon them because they feel comfortable, but you will not need darker and darker ones.

Most people should wear sunglasses for outdoor sports. They should be of the highest quality possible, but such is not always the case. An alarming number of inferior glasses are on the market and it is easy to be fooled. You should know the facts about sunglasses just as you do any other equipment you use; they are just as important.

Cheap and substandard lenses will not ruin your eyesight, unless you rely on them to absorb harmful rays and they do not. But there are risks: eyestrain, a cranky disposition, or an error in seeing, all could come from bad sunglasses and could cause you to break a leg, wreck a boat, or miss a shot.

Sunglass Density

What properties should good sunlenses have? Since the main purpose is to cut overbrightness, they must be dark, just dark enough for the conditions but no more. For average outdoor conditions, a lens should absorb 75 to 90 percent of the light which strikes it. But not just any dark lens makes a good sunglass.

One factor to consider in judging a lens is the percentage of white light absorbed. This information is supplied by the manufacturers of quality lenses. If you are unable to find out the light transmission factor of a sunlens, the manufacturer does not know or care.

The designation of lens grades is by no means uniform. Some manufacturers use an A-B-C-D system to designate degree of darkness, others use 1-2-3-4. Still others use trade names. No generally accepted standards regulate what shall be used, but you should ask for information about absorption ratios when you get sunglasses.

Exactly how dense lenses should be depends upon how you use them. Out on the water, around beach and desert, or on sunlit snow use a very dark lens, one with 85 to 90 percent absorption. For field and groundcover areas, 75 to 85 percent may be very comfortable. In forest and deep valleys, 60 to 75 percent will do. During twilight hours and on overcast days, a lens with 30 to 50 percent absorption may be adequate.

No single lens tint can handle every kind of brightness the sportsman must face. Under some conditions, any one lens tint will be either too light or too dark. Taking the lenses off if they are too dark may be the best solution as the brightness lessens. On the other hand, if yours are too light for some situations, at least they provide some glare reduction.

More than one pair? Well, ideally you could and should have lenses of different densities to deal with the varying brightness conditions you face outdoors. The next best solution is to select a lens suited to your most common need, and to learn to compensate or get along without it in other situations.

You can make a rough judgment about density by looking through the lenses in average outdoor brilliance. Give your eyes at least five minutes to adjust before you make a decision. The lenses should noticeably reduce glare, feel comfortable, yet not restrict how clearly you see.

By use of special testing equipment, the light absorption ratio of any lens can be determined. It is easy to be fooled by visual judgment alone. The color itself can make the density misleading. However, lenses which feel comfortable in any given brightness are generally adequate—though it does not follow that color is correct or that the invisible rays are blocked out.

Sunglass Tints

Just as important as how much light is absorbed by a sunlens is what kind of light. A spectrophotometer is used to determine the absorption at each wavelength and this process is important in judging the value of a lens. Reputable producers of sunglasses provide absorption curves for their lenses. You need this information to determine if lenses are effectively absorbing infrared and ultraviolet and to know the total absorption power.

The best lens is a neutral one, such as grey or smoke. A certain grey-green is also good. These lenses transmit the rays most useful in seeing and absorb those which help very little. They do not upset the normal color balance of objects seen through them.

Red, orange, blue, yellow, purple, or any bright colors are unsuitable as sunlenses. The deeper the color, the more restrictive its spectral transmission and the more it upsets the eye's normal color performance. You want none of that in the wide open spaces so stay away from the mod colors, whether delicate pastels or splashy hues.

Test sunlenses by looking through them at a white surface. Good ones should darken the surface but not make it appear appreciably colored. Try this on various colored objects. A good sunlens should not change the appearance of objects from their normal hue.

Quality of Sunglasses

Sunglasses could have acceptable darkness and color yet still be unfit to wear. The lenses should be optically pure, have no blemishes or surface spots, unwanted power, or distortions.

Check lens quality this way: Hold the lens about ten inches away. Sight on the edge of a distant picture or window frame. Slowly move the lens sidewise and notice if the image of the object jumps or waves around. With first-rate lenses, the movement will produce no effects. (This is not true of prescription lenses; image movement is expected with them.) Inspect the lenses minutely for any irregularities. Study images reflected from their surfaces. Compare the lenses to each other.

Such terms as "first quality" or "ground and polished" can be misleading, since there are no set standards or legal requirements to be met for use of these terms. Some lenses are dropped, pressed, or blown. This is a cheaper way to make them and quality is inferior. Good lenses are carefully polished and made from good optical glass or plastic to begin with.

Many believe that glass makes the finest sunlens. By adding proper ingredients, it will filter out both infrared and ultraviolet. Glass holds color and can be produced in many shades. Its optical properties are excellent, it does not scratch easily, and when heat-treated it is almost unbreakable. Most really good non-prescription sunglasses are glass.

The best assurance of quality is to seek professional advice. Rely on materials produced by reputable companies. Do not hunt for bargain, discount, or "close-out" sunglasses. Obtain sunglasses from someone who knows what he is talking about—and this is not an over-the-counter clerk who can rarely tell one lens from another.

Sunglasses should have safety lenses, especially when they are used for active sports. Your eyes are safer wearing them than with no glasses at all. Risk of eye injury is high tramping through brush, firing a gun, riding a horse, doing dozens of things. Yet millions of people perch shatterable lenses an inch from their eyeballs without giving it a second thought. Most of the first-quality sunglasses made by leading producers in the United States have break-resistant lenses.

Domestic sunglasses are generally better than foreign-made, but American manufacturers have also been known to turn out, and sell, a lot of inferior optical materials. Some imports are tolerable but it is hard to obtain scientific facts about them. So try to find out what you are buying.

Sunglass Frames

Thousands of sunglasses are unwearable because they are too small. Stay away from mini-glasses or you will see troublesome brightness contrast at the lens edge. Select a size and shape to fill your entire visual field. Face-form contours are very practical.

If the lenses are small, light can come in from the side and minimize the value of wearing them at all. Besides, the eye is attracted to the high-contrast edge. This makes it difficult to concentrate on a target, keep an eye on the ball, or even resolve the details of objects seen in the central field.

Frame fit is vital to good sunglass performance. If the bridge is too small, not only will it pinch, but it will also position the lenses too far from the face and let in too much light from the side. Short temples hurt, long ones let the frame slide down. Sunglasses, like regular glasses, are available in various dimensions, and can be selected for you. Lens density and color can also be chosen to suit your particular needs after you describe the details of your outdoor life.

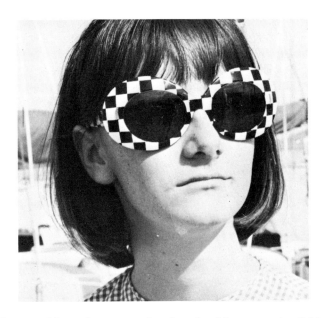

Wide frames add to glare protection but should not restrict field of view.

Few frames of any style will be comfortable without adjustment, and this is a big reason for not buying sunglasses over the counter. Besides, it is next to impossible to determine quality at supermarkets, drugstores, and gas stations. Sporting goods stores sometimes carry sunglasses made by reputable companies, but they do not provide frame adjustment.

Plastic and Polarizing Sunlenses

Plastic is also widely used for sunglass lenses. It is lightweight but scratches easily. Tints are not always stable. Plastic will not absorb ultraviolet unless especially treated and few sunlenses are. Plastic does not inhibit infrared. Good optical quality is possible in plastic but few manufacturers of sunglass lenses bother to achieve it. Mass produced sunlenses are often defective. Examine plastic lenses before purchasing. Look for imperfections, lack of uniformity. In prescription lenses, plastic is good. It is well polished, tints are controlled, and it can absorb ultraviolet.

Laminated lenses have a sheet of polarizing plastic sandwiched between two layers of glass. The polarizing material helps block reflected glare. Polarizing material is a plastic in which the chains of molecules have their axes parallel. Only light rays which are vibrating in a direction parallel to the molecules' axes will pass through the material freely. If they are vibrating ninety degrees from the molecules' axes, no light passes through. At other angles, varying amounts are transmitted, depending upon the angle.

You can easily demonstrate this with two pieces of polarizing material. Place one on top of the other and hold them toward the light. Then rotate one piece of plastic over the other; in one position little or no light passes through, while at a position oriented ninety degrees from that there is maximum transmission.

Small test pieces of material are provided with polarizing lens sunglasses to prove the lenses are truly polarizing. You could also use the two lenses themselves (if you could get them out of the frame) or two pairs of glasses. Or you can test by viewing the reflection from a shiny surface, desk, table, automobile through the polarizing lens. Rotate it as you look and see how in one position it reduces the reflection.

There is no doubt of polarizing material's ability to cut reflected light dramatically in some situations. But there are a few drawbacks. If reflected light is at the same angle as the polarizing lens is worn, no light will be absorbed and the reflection will still be there. Therefore, tilting the head changes the orientation of the polarizing factor and can let reflected glare get through. Also, inside an auto or airplane you may see disturbing patterns or stripes in safety windows—the polarizing factor detects the stress areas in the glass.

The best polarizing glass sunglasses are made with two thin layers of glass on each side of the plastic material. This makes it less subject to scratching. One glass leaf can be tinted appropriately, usually a neutral tint. The other can be used to grind a prescription. Polarizing bifocal lenses have recently been imported from Japan but as yet are not widely available.

Polarizing sunglasses of plastic are subject to the same ills as any plastic. Color must be added to the plastic and many glasses are too light.

Polarizing lenses in lightweight plastic are made in fitovers. These clip over your regular glasses and can be satisfactory for limited usage. One type handily flips up out of the way when you do not need them.

Tint-Coated and Photochromic Lenses

Lens coating can also be used to reduce the amount of light entering the eye. Coating is actually a very thin metallic layer applied to the lens surface. The density of the coating controls the amount of light reduction. The color of the coating determines which wave lengths are blocked. By combination of color and density, almost any kind of selective light transmission is possible with coating.

A unique value of coating is the gradient density effect. The metallic film can be added so as to shade from dense at the top, to light at the bottom of the lens. This works well to provide maximum protection from high overhead brightness.

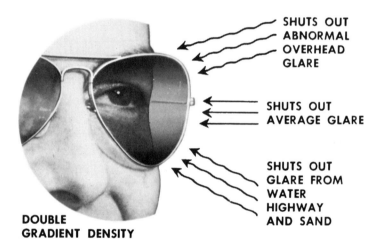

SHUTS OUT ABNORMAL OVERHEAD GLARE

SHUTS OUT AVERAGE GLARE

SHUTS OUT GLARE FROM WATER HIGHWAY AND SAND

DOUBLE GRADIENT DENSITY

Coated double gradient density lenses have maximum glare protection at top and bottom, permit more light through the central seeing area. (Courtesy of Bausch & Lomb)

Double gradient density lenses are also available. They shade from dark at top and bottom to lighter in the middle. This has a use outdoors where glare is excessive from sky above and water or snow below, yet a light area of the lens center is needed to look straight ahead or work around a vehicle.

A special lens recently developed has intriguing advantages for

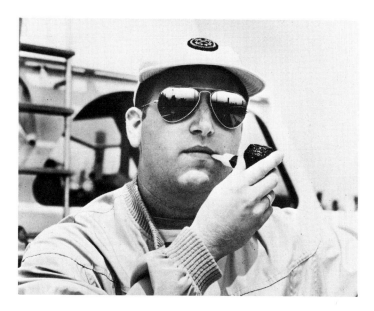

Note that on these gradient sunglasses there is great reflection from the top of the lenses and very little from the bottom. They therefore offer maximum glare protection from sky brightness. *(Courtesy of Bausch & Lomb)*

sportsmen. This is photochromic glass, which automatically adjusts to the amount of light. Outdoors the lens darkens, inside it clears. It is available in·neutral gray and in prescription lenses, including bifocals.

Actually the photochromic lens is not a sunglass and the manufacturer does not claim it is one. Depending upon temperature and amount of sunlight, the lens at maximum will absorb 50 to 60 percent of the light, not enough to put it in the true sunglass range. Still, for some people who do not need a dark lens or want to bother with two pairs, it is very useful. Its speed of adjustment is adequate and the process exhibits no fatigue or deterioration.

The photochromic lens can be made more useful for the outdoorsman by adding a very light coating to the neutral gray tint. With a 15 to 25 percent reflective coating applied to the back surface, the lens absorbs only 30 to 40 percent in its lightest phase yet blocks out 70 to 80 percent at maximum density. Thus, it would adjust to the amount of light during the day over a useful range.

Coatings are added only on special order to photochromic lenses.

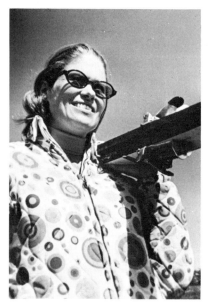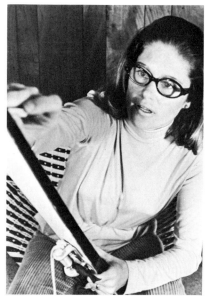

Photochromic lenses, known as Photogray, are virtually clear indoors, but outside they darken. However, they never turn quite as dark as true sunglasses. *(Courtesy of Corning Glass Works)*

Be sure that the coating is not too dark or the variability range will become too compressed. A bad feature of this lens is that it cannot function inside a car, boat, or plane since it depends on ultraviolet light to make its change and this is filtered out by windows.

Sunglasses in Prescription

If you wear a correction for distance seeing, you should have prescription sunglasses. Since you can only get them from a professional man, all the uncertainties of quality, tint, size and so on are eliminated. But be sure to describe your outdoor needs in detail (how you hunt, fish, golf, or water ski) so he can prescribe most accurately—not only tint but lens power as well.

Prescription lenses come in a large variety of tints and densities, both in glass and plastic. Complicated lenses and multifocals (bifocals and trifocals) can be made in most colors. Indeed, bifocal wearers need them in sunglasses to do a variety of tasks from reading maps to tying a fly.

Costs of prescription sunglasses are hard to predict since there are so many variables in both lenses and frames and in the services that must go with them. Besides, there is the cost of the vision examination. Fees also differ throughout the country and between practitioners. Do not look for bargains. You should have the best professional services and the finest materials, just as you would want when you purchase any outdoor equipment.

Clip-on sunlenses can be worn with prescription glasses. Some are quite good, others bad. A problem arises since regular glasses are generally smaller than sunglasses should be. Weight is also a problem with clip-ons, as are the reflections from the extra surfaces of the fitover. For limited usage, however, fitovers may prove satisfactory.

Contact lens wearers have two choices. Contacts, being plastic, can be tinted like any plastic and are subject to the same pros and cons. For long hours outdoors, contact lenses in suntint are very convenient. For going in and out, frequent removal and change of lenses is a nuisance. For that reason, some wearers prefer the second choice: plain sunglasses used with contacts.

Some Recommendations

For men: Fortunately, sunglasses for men have long been made large and rugged. Quality varies but those designed particularly for sportsmen are high grade. The aviator-type metal goggle, driving glasses in a large plastic frame, even some plastic shields and ski goggles are good choices. Seek sound advice for special items—sunglasses can be made in most any form you wish.

For women: Stay away from the extremes, too large and too small, and from cosmetic specs for use outdoors; these are usually tinted too lightly for adequate glare protection. High cost here does not always mean quality—it may be for style not lenses. On the other hand, excellent sunglasses are made in the latest fashions; be sure they fit well and cover your field of view. Most of the sunglass junk is designed to attract the woman buyer.

For children: Visual scientists are not sure why young children seldom require glare protection. They often want sunglasses to emulate adults, and there is really no reason they should not wear them. Their need seems to become greater as they get into the teens. Safety lenses are a must and plastic is adequate for children's needs.

chapter **10**

using

optical

aids

The eye often needs help for outdoor sports. Even the most normal eyes can benefit from image magnification to see better for hunting, boating, bird watching, or enjoying a spectator sport. Binoculars, telescopes, or sport glasses have long been used to add accuracy and enjoyment to seeing outdoors.

There is a great deal more to this matter of binoculars and telescopes than will be covered here. Optics, quality, cost, construction, and design should be carefully considered before you choose any optical aids for your use. There are a number of good books on the subject—study one until you know enough to make an informed selection.

This chapter will consider only the visual factors involved in using magnification devices, not the mechanics of the devices themselves. You will do a much better job not only selecting but also using binoculars or telescopic devices if you understand how they relate to your vision needs for outdoor tasks.

Need for Magnification

When is magnification needed, whether by binoculars, monoculars, or a fancy telescope? The answer is: at any time when you cannot see as sharply as you would like to because the image is too small—a frequent happening outdoors even if your eyes have normal visual acuity.

Naturally if the eye does not have good visual acuity, the need for magnified images is even greater. So if vision is not normal, binoculars are particularly necessary. Since visual acuity tends to lessen with age, this means everyone may eventually benefit from magnification for seeing tasks that could formerly have been done with ease.

Binoculars

It is true that use of binoculars will make up for minor errors of refraction of the eye, although using them is not recommended as a solution. However, if you need only a small lens correction yet choose not to wear glasses because they get in the way behind the binoculars, the magnification produced by the binoculars can offset the slightly blurred vision you might otherwise have. (The trouble is that your vision gets help only while you're looking through the magnification device.)

Now it is also true that the eyepieces of many binoculars and telescopes can be adjusted to compensate for visual errors. There is a limit though and most cannot correct more than two diopters or so of error. This is a rather small amount and less than many people who are dependent upon glasses are likely to have.

The other limit to compensating for a visual error by eyepiece adjustment is that only spherical errors can be corrected. Small amounts of nearsightedness and farsightedness can be handled by proper eyepiece settings in most good magnification devices—binoculars, telescopes, rifle scopes, and even microscopes. But they cannot be adjusted for astigmatism. Its correction takes a special kind of lens and one oriented in a certain position, and such an arrangement cannot be satisfactorily built into an adjustable eyepiece.

To some degree, certain kinds of astigmatism can be compensated for by spherical lenses. It may be possible to see fairly well with the spherical equivalent of the compound lens required to correct astigmatism. This is a matter of selecting a spherical lens, either concave (minus) or convex (plus) which will produce the best focus instead of the cylindrical lens system necessary to produce perfect imagery.

Try it and see. Adjust the eyepiece, even though you do have a small degree of astigmatism, to the best possible focus. As a matter of fact, certain types of astigmatism even in higher degrees can be corrected quite well with spherical equivalents. If the image seems clear enough to suit you through the binoculars, that is all that is necessary. The spherical equivalent lens would never do for regular wear, you would be too uncomfortable. But for the limited time you look through binoculars, you should have little problem.

Whether you need magnification also obviously depends upon what you are trying to do. It is not very rewarding to study the moon with the unaided eye. On the other hand, a celestial telescope is hardly needed to locate a pheasant in a cornfield. The kind of need is of fundamental importance in selecting binoculars or telescopes—you must consider whether magnification should be large or small, what size of field will be most useful, and how bright the image need be.

Individual requirements vary as well. Some individuals with good visual acuity and normal seeing responses seem to require more magnification than others, or some magnification when others do not. Psychological factors may be involved, but these are as yet unanalyzed by visual scientists. Other people are annoyed by the reduced field of view through field glasses and the interference the lenses, the tubes, and the objectives represent. So where one person will reach for binoculars another will disdain them completely.

Experience in how to use binoculars properly may be a reason for these differences. So may be the ability to spot things and recognize details, based upon the many factors of visual performance described in Chapter 4. Training, experience, speed of recognition, eye movement efficiency, and perceptual skills may be greater in the person who does not need a boost in image size.

If you feel the need to use binoculars a great deal, this does not necessarily indicate any particular visual problem. And there is no reason not to use them since they do not hurt your eyes or create any dependence. Even very bad binoculars cannot damage eyesight, although momentary discomfort might result.

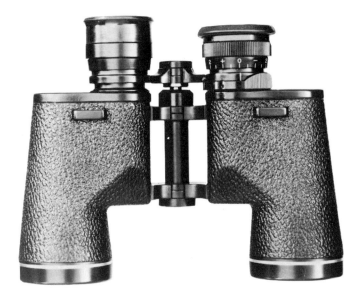

Right eyepiece on these binoculars is adjustable to compensate for small visual errors. The markings are in diopters, the plus side correcting far-sightedness, the minus side nearsightedness. The soft rubber cup on the right eyepiece has been rolled back for use with sunglasses or regular eyeglasses. *(Courtesy Bushnell Optical Corporation)*

Neither is there any particular type of binocular or telescope, or power ratio or field size that solves a visual problem better than another. These devices should be chosen for the job they are to do rather than to fit the eyes of the user. The possible exception is that if a person's corrected visual acuity is less than normal, he may require magnification a little greater than normal.

Wearing Glasses While Using Binoculars

Since this book strongly recommends that every outdoorsman have glasses—at least sunglasses and, for many uses, safety lenses—the problems of wearing glasses and looking through eyepieces should confront everyone. It is obviously easier to see through eyepieces of binoculars and telescopes without glasses in the way, since the eye must be placed at just one point to see the largest field the optical system is capable of producing, and to get the sharpest focus possible throughout that field. This one point is called the *eyepoint*. Located behind the back surface of the ocular lens (the lens of the eyepiece), it can be found by moving a translucent screen (a piece of waxed paper will do) back and forth behind the eyepieces while the binoculars are directed at a bright distant object. Note when the circular image is sharpest and brightest. It is usually about half an inch (thirteen millimeters) from the surface of the eyepiece lens.

The pupil of the eye (actually the center of the entrance pupil of the eye) must be placed at the eyepoint. The center of the pupil of the eye lies a little over three millimeters behind the front surface of the cornea. Thus, if the eyepoint is about one-half inch or thirteen millimeters, a space of only ten millimeters is left between the back surface of the eyepiece lens and the front of the cornea of the eye. Some of this space must be filled with hardware.

Spectacle lenses and frames are designed to fit so that the lenses lie in a plane thirteen millimeters from the front of the cornea. In actual practice, this is rarely achieved and the distance tends to be greater rather than less. Also, lens thickness varies and tends to cut down further on the available eyepoint space. Because of this, the eyepoint would have to be greater than half an inch from the binocular lens surface when wearing eyeglass lenses; otherwise the viewer could not get close enough to see the entire field of view even if his spectacles were tight against the back surface of the eyepiece lens.

None of this makes any allowance for thickness of the casing which holds the binocular eyepiece lens or of the eyecup, which is usually designed to shield the eye from peripheral glare. Add as much as a quarter of an inch, up to six millimeters, for this necessary hardware and it is easy to understand the impossibility of looking through ordinary eyepieces while wearing glasses and getting the full field. One solution is to press the spectacles closer to the eye. This may not be physically possible but if it is, the spectacle lens itself will no longer be in its proper position and delivering the right power.

A better solution is to purchase binoculars (or telescopes) especially designed to permit wearing glasses. Some have rubber eyecups which can be pressed forward so the pupil of the eye can get close to the eyepoint (though this is rarely accomplished if the eye-point is short.) Eyecups on these instruments are short or fold over and have the advantage of giving good glare protection when used without glasses.

Some binoculars have practically no eyecups, and what does exist is made very flat. It is also helpful if the optical system is built so

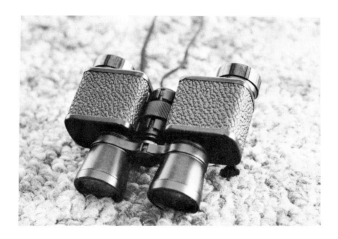

This compact 8 x 25 binoculars has flat eyepieces to permit easy viewing while wearing glasses.

that the eyepoint is farther back, three-quarters of an inch or more. Eyepoints of telescopic rifle sights are much longer, for reasons to be covered later, but their field of view is also very small.

A good way to determine if the eyepoint of a device is suitable for wearing glasses is to try it. Look through any binoculars or tele-scope, and by moving your eye closer or farther, determine the largest field of view that is visible. Notice objects at the edge of the field so you can compare width while wearing glasses. Repeat the field size test with lenses on. Chances are that even crowding as close as you can get, the field size will be less. It is practically impossible to get close enough to the eyepoint while wearing glasses to get the full field, and unfortunately this is true of binoculars designed to use with eyeglasses.

The problems of leaving glasses on suggest they be taken off when using binoculars. There are advantages, and getting to the eyepoint is the main one of them. Whether it is practical or not depends upon

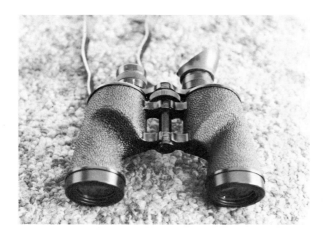

Right eyepiece here has a broad rubber side shield which is excellent for blocking out light from the side. It can be rolled down for use with eyeglasses, but even then it is impossible to get to the eyepoint.

the amount of lens prescription that is in the spectacles and how much can be compensated by adjusting the binocular eyepiece. Without glasses, there are fewer lenses surfaces to look through and this increases image brightness a little.

What if you are wearing sunglasses then take them off to look through binoculars in bright daylight? Generally you will have no problem. The binoculars have a small field, the eyepieces shield the eyes and the total amount of light is greatly reduced. If there are wide eyecups, especially the broad rubber ones, the side glare is cut out and seeing can be very comfortable. But for pure convenience, it is handier to leave spectacles in place, provided the eyepoint distance permits seeing the entire field.

Power Factor of Magnifying Devices

Why all the concern about eyepoint? Is not magnification more important? The answer depends upon what the binoculars are to be used for. There is a limit to the power needed for general sports use. The eye needs more information than is brought to it by a huge image. As power increases, width of field decreases and image brightness lessens. Then too, beyond a certain magnification, generally 10-power, it is impossible to hand-hold the device without annoying image movement.

The power needed depends upon what the field glasses are to be used for. A 5-power increases the image five times its normal size, or 500 percent. The step from a 5-power to 10-power only doubles the image, thus is only a 100 percent increase. The increase from a 5-power to a 7-power is only 40 percent. Increasing power boosts image size at a decreasing rate and it has to be decided whether the added magnification is worth the problems it creates.

Field Size and Good Vision

Field size itself may not be of great importance. For studying the details of an object, identifying a bird, or spotting a shot group on a target, magnification is needed but the field does not have to be large. Following the movements of a grizzly working his way up a slope or watching the fast action of a football game requires good field size. Only the very center of a field has to be sharp in order to study detail. All that is needed to match the human eye is a one-degree central area. That is the size of the fovea, the tiny central spot of the retina packed with cones which provide the sharpest visual acuity the eye possesses.

A scope with sharp imagery in a central one degree area could be used just like the eye if the scope were moved around to center on objects. Of course this suggestion is not practical—rather, the eye moves around to look through the area provided by the scope or binoculars—but it does illustrate that field size for some purposes can be very small. And it also explains why the field is better if it is sharp to the very edge (requiring fine optics), because the glasses need not be moved so much to maintain sharp imagery.

If your binoculars have some field defects such as curvature of field or spherical aberration, these can be compensated for somewhat by moving them around and looking more through the centers. Still better, get good optics in the first place. However, field does have value. It is natural to center an image in the field; to a degree this helps the viewer to relate the image to its background and adds to its meaning.

Binoculars or scopes used for searching should have a wide field—the wider the better. Once an object is located it can be examined in

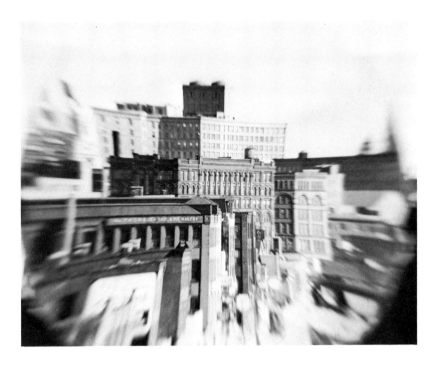

Curvature of the field—a common defect of cheap binoculars with inferior optics. Only the central area of the lens system is clear here; the periphery is very distorted. *(Courtesy of Bausch & Lomb. © 1970 Popular Science Publishing Co.)*

the central field. This is the way the eyes themselves work. One advantage of zoom power systems is that low power and wide field are available for locating, then greater power, though the field becomes small, for inspection.

A wide objective lens allows more light to enter and improves image brightness, and some binoculars are made with wide objectives so they are useful in dim light. However, the field size is determined by both the focal length of the objective lenses and the diameter of the eyepiece.

Field size is generally expressed as so many feet at 1000 yards. When the field is said to be 300 feet it means that the width of the real field is 300 feet in diameter at a distance of 1000 yards from the binoculars. Field can also be stated in degrees. One degree at 1000 yards is about 52 feet. So a field of five degrees has a diameter of about 260 feet 1000 yards away. Fields of from five to ten degrees are common in binoculars, often being somewhere in the middle of that range, and these serve well to accomplish what is needed.

Apparent field size is also important. This is the angular distance through which the eye would have to move in order to look from one edge of the field to the other. If it is large, it adds a certain sense of reality to looking through field glasses, a sort of I'm-right-there feeling. In an intangible way, it may add a little to accurate perception.

The apparent field can be calculated by multiplying the angular field of a system by the magnifying power. For example, if the real angular field is seven degrees (or about 364 feet at 1000 yards) and the power is 7, the apparent field is forty-nine degrees. The eyes normally can move through about one hundred degrees laterally but only about two thirds of that is "usable" before head movements are made. The apparent field width is from forty to sixty degrees for "standard" binoculars. A high-power spotting scope can have an apparent field as large as or larger than ordinary binoculars even though its real field is very small.

Brightness of the Image

The ability of an optical system to transmit light is determined in some degree by the quality of its optics. Naturally this will affect the sharpness of the image as well. There may be as many as eight to ten lenses and four to six prisms in a good pair of binoculars. All must be of high quality and carefully matched and mounted. Like other quality products, better optical systems cost more but deliver more and are generally worth the expense.

Image brightness is also affected by the use of coating on the lens surfaces. Without it, as much as 5 to 6 percent of the incident light can be lost by reflection at each lens surface. This can mount up to a 50 percent loss in an entire system having eight to ten surfaces. Coating reduces the loss to some 3 percent per surface. The resultant gain in image brightness can be very significant. The better binoculars and telescopes have high quality coating on all optical surfaces.

A third factor in determining image brightness is the size of the exit pupil. This is the optically created limiting aperture size through which all rays leaving the systems must pass. You can see the exit pupils very easily by holding binoculars a foot or so away from you directed at a bright surface and by noting the bright discs produced by the eyepieces—they seem to float in air a short distance behind the eyepiece. The size can be figured by dividing the objective diameter by the power factor. For example, a 7 × 35 pair of binoculars has exit pupils which are five millimeters in diameter.

The diameter of the exit pupil need be no larger than the diameter of the pupil of the viewing eye. If it is, some of the light is going to waste and is not entering the eye anyway. In ordinary outdoor daylight viewing conditions, the diameter of the human pupil is 2.5 to 3.0 millimeters. Behind the binoculars the pupils may dilate to 4 millimeters. So a 6 × 25 or 7 × 26 provides a large enough exit pupil to match the eye. The very popular 7 × 35 produces a 5-millimeter exit pupil which is adequate even in some less bright conditions. A 7 × 50 produces a 7.1 exit pupil which is the maximum size to which the pupil of the eye can dilate.

The 7 × 50 designation means of course that the power of the instrument is 7, it magnifies 7 times. The 50 is the diameter of the objective lens in millimeters. It partially tells how bright the image will be, since with these two figures the exit pupil size can easily be calculated. Some manufacturers use a light efficiency rating to express the image brightness. But not all provide this information and so it is difficult to make valid comparisons.

Using Two Eyes with Binoculars

There is no point in using binoculars unless you have binocular vision. If you do, it is normal to use them because using two eyes is more natural and more comfortable; two eyes provide a wider overall field, and there is some enhancement of depth perception. But try closing one eye and compare how things look this way with the view obtained by both eyes. The difference is not really so great as you might expect.

A person who has good vision in only one eye, whose eyes do not coordinate, or who has a tendency to suppress one eye's image, may as well use a monocular. Even for the individual with normal two-eyed seeing, a monocular will produce nearly the same results as a binocular. The biggest drawback is the necessity of closing one eye. This may be a nuisance. If you can do it easily, you can save money and get along with a much more compact magnifying device. Nevertheless, monoculars are much less popular than binoculars, possibly because vision just does not seem quite so natural with them.

Some people have trouble looking through binoculars because it is difficult for their eyes to fuse the two images. This is a so-called muscle fusion problem and was covered in Chapter 3. When looking into the tubes of a binocular sighting device, the fusional process of such eyes is so disturbed that it is impossible to hold the images single. The result is double vision, which can be corrected either by exercises or by prism glasses. Otherwise the best bet is to use a monocular.

Binoculars must be kept in perfect alignment or the image may appear blurred or doubled. Small amounts of misalignment are difficult to detect, creating only a vague sense of discomfort—a feeling that things are "not looking just right." In a well-made optical instrument the lenses are mounted better than in cheaper models and can take rough handling. Misalignment can be checked by sighting on a small distant object. The binoculars should be fixed in position, laid flat, and weighted down or held by any method to maintain stability. Move the binoculars until the test object appears just at the edge of one field, for example at the extreme left side. Check with one eye at a time, alternately closing one and then the other. The object should hold the same position near the edge with either eye. Try it with the object in other positions, such as 9, 12, 3, and 6 o'clock.

The eyes themselves can compensate for small amounts of misalignment, at least for brief periods of time and especially if the displacement is lateral. But vertical or rotational displacement can seriously interfere with seeing properly.

Individual eyepiece adjustments are handy in case the two eyes differ slightly. These would not be necessary if glasses are worn while using binoculars, since through the corrective lenses the eye should have no refractive error. If you find it necessary to consistently adjust the eyepieces for best imagery, either the binoculars themselves are off (possibly the scale setting is incorrect) or your glasses need changing.

It is more comfortable and more normal to look through binoculars if the optical centers of the two eyepieces are exactly the same distance apart as the centers of the optical systems of the viewer's eyes. If they are not, prismatic effects can be created, producing double vision and distortion. The separation of the centers of the eyepieces should be equal to the interpupillary distance of the eyes when sighting on a distant object. This is the distance between the centers of the pupils and is easily measured when your eyes are examined. Ask what your PD (interpupillary distance) is. That way you can get the exact setting for your binoculars. Eyes range in separation from about fifty-five to seventy-five millimeters, with the great majority falling in the sixties. Most binoculars provide for an adjustment range from about fifty-eight to seventy. A scale is provided on the center post to indicate the eyepiece separation.

If you do not know what your interpupillary distance is in millimeters, you will have to adjust binoculars to a "what seems best" separation. Move the eyepieces closer together or farther apart while looking through them until the individual fields blend into a single field. They may not appear as one completely circular field; rather one a little wider than it is high. But it will be a comfortable and normal-appearing field. Things will "look right." Note the setting on the tube separation scale, adjust to this same setting each time you use the binoculars.

Many of the principles already discussed apply to other kinds of optical aids—a complex telescope, a simple sport magnifier, a loupe, or almost any compound optical system. Quality of material and workmanship are paramount considerations. If they are top grade, the optics are bound to be good. But it is easy to be misled by high-powered advertising which preys on the ignorance of the purchaser. Frequently, the bigger the ad and the louder its claims, the more misleading it is—especially when "high quality optics" are advertised for a very low price.

Gunsights

A very common use of optical aid for outdoors is a telescopic sight. They have advantages over open and aperture sights for long range, accurate sighting in rifle shooting and even in pistol shooting. However, many shooters will argue that they can produce great results with ordinary sights—and they can.

The purpose here is not to evaluate the many pros and cons of gunsights. There are excellent books on this subject. But just as with binoculars, certain visual factors need to be considered. Read what follows keeping this in mind.

Gunsights come in many designs all intended to improve aligning accuracy. There is no absolute proof of which style is best—bright-

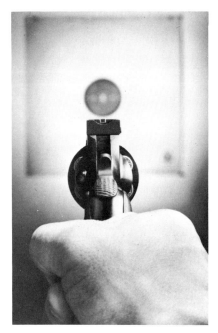 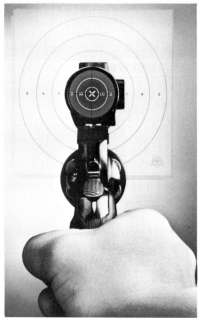

Left: View over open pistol sights; front sight is clear, distant target is blurred.
Right: With telescopic sight, the distant target is clear as well as the cross-hairs of the scope. *(Courtesy of the Bushnell Optical Corporation)*

ness and target background all enter into the picture. The eye's most delicate aligning ability is in detecting a break in a vertical line. The eye can do this, under good conditions, down to one second of arc accuracy. But sighting devices do not rely on this principle alone; some depend upon the ability to judge the width of interspaces, while others use a type of aligning and centering function. This is very much like a measure of visual acuity. Thus it is obvious that the better the natural acuity of the eye, the more accurate sighting can be.

Cross-hair sights are based upon the centering function of the eye in some degree but more on an alignment process—getting the target in alignment with the fine cross hairs. The great advantage of the cross hair is that it readily provides instant information on alignment, both vertical and horizontal, yet the cross hairs themselves are almost invisible.

Open and Aperture Gunsights

Open sights are actually not an aid to vision but rather an aid to aiming. With open sights, full correction of vision is essential. Keep in mind too that as age gallops along, vision that could once draw a perfect bead with the front sight probably needs some help. This is inevitably true for the pistol shooter, and special visual aid may be necessary, as covered in Chapter 11.

Aperture sights are, in a way, an aid to vision, particularly if the peephole is held close to the eye, as it can be in low caliber firearms. This can be demonstrated by looking through a very small opening at a distant object. Make a pinhole (a rather large one) in a cardboard. Hold this close to an eye with an uncorrected refractive error (for myopia it works especially well) and the result is sharpened vision. Aperture sights tend to do the same thing. The smaller the aperture, the less light enters the eye, but the optical effect is greater, until the hole becomes too small. It is also important to consider the size of the field you want to see through the opening. Field depends upon projection distance as well as how far the opening is from the eye. (Size of the rear sight opening depends upon the size and type of front sight used.) But the aperture sight should not be selected to aid vision—corrective glasses are better—but rather for its qualities as an aligning device.

One of the drawbacks of open and aperture sights is that they block part of the target. This is especially true of open sights, which can cover the lower half of a deer. When shooting target on range, it matters little whether or not the entire pattern can be seen but when shooting live animals it does make a difference. From a visual standpoint, the more of the target that can be seen, the better will be its identification and, in some degree, the more accurate the aiming, particularly with moving game. Aperture sights also block out some of the target.

Most aperture sights are too small. There is no reason they need be small as long as the front-sight centering system is a good one. Naturally there is an upper limit; it is impossible to center a pinhead in a three-foot circle. But if the opening is too small, the eye cannot get into the proper position to move the front sight into alignment.

A small aperture is good for deliberate long-range aiming when the rifle barrel can be rested on something. A large one is easier to use on moving targets. To meet a varying range of conditions, an adjustable iris type aperture is made, which has advantages. Another way to suit varying visual demands is to use several aperture sizes, changing them appropriately according to the lighting and the kind of shooting.

Telescopic Gunsights

The telescope is a significant optical aid because of the magnified image it produces. Rays of light leaving the ocular surface of the eyepiece are parallel. As far as the eye is concerned, these rays come from optical infinity and there is no problem of focusing on the front sight of either a rifle or a pistol, as often is the case with open or aperture sights. This feature alone makes the telescopic sight the best choice for the shooter whose eye has lost its near-focusing ability (presbyopia). With a telescopic device the reticule is clear and so is the target, once the scope has been adjusted to the shooter's eye (following the manufacturer's instructions).

The cross-hair reticule is an accurate aligning mechanism, as has already been pointed out. When viewing a field of any size at all (and most are reasonably large), one gets no partial blocking of the target; for moving game and quick sighting, the telescopic sight is excellent. The eyepiece of a telescopic sight, like that of binoculars, can be adjusted to compensate for certain visual errors.

But, as has been said, glasses with safety lenses should be worn for all shooting. Since glasses are to be worn, they can carry any necessary lens prescription, although there is a cost factor to consider. It may prove less expensive to wear plain safety lenses and adjust the telescopic sight's eyepiece to correct the eye's minor refractive errors than to have prescription lenses made and changed frequently. The decision could depend upon how badly a visual correction is needed when not using the scope.

Eye Relief

Sights which extend above the rifle barrel, as do peep sights and all telescopics, must have adequate eye relief. Like the eyepoint of binoculars, eye relief is the distance from the telescopic scope's eyepiece at which the eye must be to get the full field of view. The situation is not the same for an aperture sight which has no optics involved; in that case, moving closer does increase the field of view. Eye relief distance does give the eye "relief," by providing room for

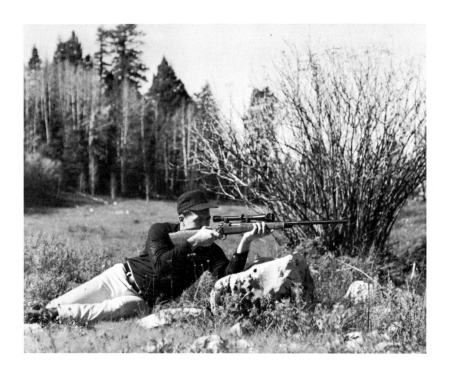

Notice the eye relief. Enough room must be left between the back of the scope and the eye to prevent injury when the gun recoils. *(Courtesy of the W. R. Weaver Company)*

the firearm to recoil at discharge without the hardware of the sight smashing into the face.

How much eye relief is necessary depends upon the gun's caliber, how tightly the stock is held to the shoulder, and whether or not the eye is actually held at the correct distance. More properly, the vital distance is the eyebrow relief—the distance from the back edge of the telescopic sight tube (the surface of the eyepiece lens is always inside the tube rim a short distance) to the eyebrow (which extends forward in front of the pupil of the eye). Obviously the eyebrow relief is shorter than the eye relief.

Wearing glasses will lessen the relief distance. Eyeglasses may project forward of the eyebrow line. If any convincing is necessary that all shooting glasses should have safety lenses, think of the tube of a telescopic eyepiece slamming toward glass lenses at high impact. There seems to be no standard agreement by manufacturers as to whether the eye relief quoted for their telescopic sights is actually eyebrow relief, or the true, optically correct eyepoint. For high powered rifles, it should be 3 inches. Those on the market range from about 2¼ to 3¾ inches.

Some scopes can be adjusted to suit the individual's aiming habits. Certain shooters crowd forward on the stock and need the sight adjusted forward accordingly. With aperture sights, the shooter must be careful not to move inside the eye relief distance, although he could do this without affecting the aiming process. Find out the eyebrow relief of the scope you use. You cannot always rely on the manufacturer's figures; some tend to mislead in this regard. Sight normally and have someone measure the distance. If you must sight closer than a safe relief distance for the gun's recoil do something about it— move back to a safe distance even though it reduces field or get another scope.

Power and Field Size of Telescopic Sights

Power and field size relate to each other the same way in telescopic sights as in binoculars. Magnification is not everything. On the other hand, field size is not of great importance in the actual aiming process, especially for target shooting. Field size is significant, however, in the locating process, such as finding the varmint in the sights. Field size for telescopic sights is specified as the diameter in feet of the field at 100 yards (not 1000 yards as used for binocular field sizes). Field widths on typical telescopic sights range from as small as 10 to 12 feet on 10-power scopes, to 50 feet on 2-power.

For close range shooting and working in brush country, a 2- to 3-power scope is recommended. It gives a wide field and can be used to follow a moving target. The eyes need their peripheral fields to follow and locate targets. Medium-distance shooting for general purpose use is generally best done with a 4- to 5-power. The field is smaller but at the distance at which it is used, the shooter is less likely to fire at a moving target.

A 6- to 7-power scope is considered best for medium- to long-

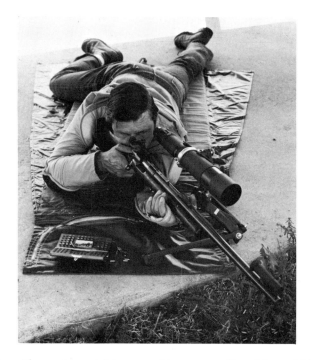

Especially with aperture sights, a spotting scope, like this variable 15- to 60-power model, is needed to see shot placement. *(Courtesy of the Redfield Gun Sight Co.)*

range use in open country. The field is small and firing is done only at stationary targets. In the 8- to 9-power range and beyond in the 10- to 12-power, it is almost impossible to steady the rifle except in prone positions or using a rest. Variable-power scopes can extend through a range of as much as 8 powers. Certainly one factor to consider, besides the usual standards of magnification for firing distance and the type of hunting, is the best visual acuity of the hunter's eye. When sensitivity of the eye drops, it may be wise to choose a slightly stronger power.

Telescopic sights are sometimes used to identify game, to know if it is male or female, legal size or not, or, for that matter, to detect whether the object is man or beast! Unequivocal identification is so essential it hardly needs saying. Many of the suggestions in this book will aid visual performance and in object identification outdoors. The

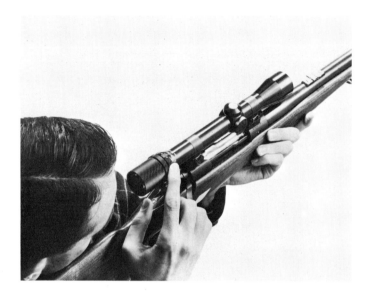

Some telescopic rifle sights have a sighting post which can be flipped into position when darkness prevents seeing the cross-hairs. This feature can add a great deal to visibility of the sighting mechanism and can increase accuracy. *(Courtesy of the Bushnell Optical Corporation)*

telescopic sight may make it easier in some cases—but it also creates a rather curious situation.

Suppose you were a hunter, wearing blaze orange as you should, and discovered you were being studied by another hunter through the scope sight of his 30-06. He is trying to make out if you have horns or not. The safety is still on but his finger hangs idly on the trigger. The light is bad. You blend with the background. At long range he is not really sure what you are.

That situation may be far better than where the hunter was guessing without the help of magnification. But somehow you might feel a little more comfortable if the telescope did not have a rifle attached.

part **three**

vision
in
sports

chapter 11

vision for
hunting and
marksmanship

Everyone should wear glasses when shooting. Yes, *everyone*. Every-one who wants complete eye protection and the best vision pos-sible no matter what the shooting condition, to say nothing of comfort and pleasure from eyes which perform at peak efficiency. Naturally anyone with fuzzy vision should wear corrective lenses when stepping to the firing line or on the hunting grounds, but there are reasons why marksmen and hunters with perfect sight should wear glasses as well.

The most important reason is eye protection. Many guns toss enough debris back out of the chamber when a shell is fired to present hazard of eye injury. Twigs flip into the eyes when hunters are scrambling through the brush, they can fall on rough ground and shatter ordinary glass spectacles—even ordinary handling and pack-ing when out in the field can cause lens breakage.

As stated in Chapter 6, a lens should be three-millimeter case-hardened glass or made of plastic to be safest from the impact it may

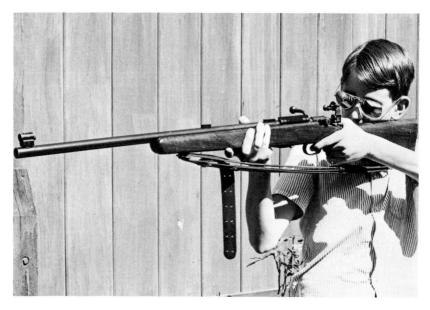

Glasses should be worn whenever firing a gun—safety glasses. Youngsters should learn this early.

have to take while worn for hunting or shooting target. Have any shooting glasses you use made for safety. Most of the shooting glasses sold in the United States by reputable manufacturers have break-resistant lenses. If they do not, don't buy them.

What has been said about sunglasses in Chapter 9 applies here. Glare protection is certainly necessary for hunting and is needed many times also on the firing range. Sunglasses should be large and dark enough, and by all means should be safety lenses.

A very common tint made for shooting glasses is a bright yellow. These lenses are not sunglasses but do cut the intensity of incident light slightly. A yellow lens or any tinted lens will do this somewhat, though it may not seem to when you look through it. The yellow may also create the effect of making objects appear brighter, but no lens can "gather light," or increase the amount entering the eye. The yellow lens then cannot improve seeing when worn at night—as some claims would have it do.

Yellow lenses, at least those scientifically compounded, tend to reduce the veiling effect of ultraviolet and infrared wavelengths. They absorb the blue and cut down the scatter light of fog and haze. Certainly yellow filters sharpen photographs taken in hazy atmosphere, but the eye does not have the same sensitivity as a photographic emulsion. Still, yellow does apparently increase object visibility somewhat, although it must be said that research has failed to prove conclusively what the real value of wearing yellow lenses is, if indeed there is any.

A theoretical explanation of yellow's sharpening effect is based upon a reduction of the chromatic spread of focus in the eye. This no doubt happens in some small degree, but it does not happen equally in all eyes. The spectrum narrowing may in some cases increase the contrast of a bull's-eye on its white background but apparently this effect is related to the subject's feeling about it as much as to anything else. Some people feel yellow is very beneficial, some can tell no difference, while others report that it is disturbing and causes headaches.

In any case, yellow is primarily of value for range shooting and when the atmosphere is grey and hazy. In the field, yellow should not be used on bright, clear days. Yellow colors everything yellow and minimizes the value of color vision; under some circumstances, certain eyes may consider this an advantage in spotting game while others will find it a handicap.

Special Frames for Shooting

Lens color and safety are not the only factors to consider in selecting shooting glasses that are right for you. Even the ideal lens must be positioned perfectly in front of your eye; it must be the right size to give maximum protection. This takes a frame that fits your features so comfortably that you scarcely notice its presence on your face.

For any type of hunting and for skeet and trap shooting, spectacle frames should provide maximum visibility of the entire visual field. To spot game or clay bird instantly, eyes must sweep a large area before the head has time to turn frames out of the way. Frames should conform to facial contours and set high enough to make aiming possible through the upper portion of the lens. This is one reason that "everyday" prescription frames or sunglasses probably will not do for shooting. Check your line of vision in aiming position when selecting a frame; be sure you can see without obstruction.

Frames used for shooting must be precisely adjusted to your own facial characteristics. The lenses must be angled correctly and at the proper distance for your eyes. The lens slant has something to do with its optical effects. If it is too close to the face, it can fog and steam up; if too far away, it will let in too much light around the corners.

For target shooting with rifle and pistol, size is less important, except for the factor of glare at the edge. Indoors even this does not matter. However, there is no reason the frame should be small; the visibility of the lens rim may create a psychological interference. Any shooting glasses should be, therefore, larger than average.

Selection of proper type and length of temple (earpiece) is essential also. The skull type temples fit tightly to the head, angle behind the ear, and are comfortable but less secure than the wraparound metal type. For rough going, wraparounds may be better; for target the skull type may be quite adequate. But what counts most is proper fitting; the length must be correct in the first place, then the temple bent to hold snugly without being too tight.

Lens shape and its position on the face are especially important for shooting. Large face-form shapes are good in providing a wide field of view and eliminating glare around the edge; however, they may not be positioned properly when sighting. Since the head is tilted down, the line of sight passes high in the lens and unless the frame is set high on the face, the frame edge can get in the way.

Metal frames, or plastic and metal combinations with adjustable pads have advantages for shooting. With such frames, the pads can be adjusted to set the lens higher if need be. Plastic frames with a fixed bridge may work if bridge size and lens shape is appropriate. How high the lens will be positioned depends also upon the individual's anatomy—the position of eyes in relation to bridge of nose, and how prominent the bridge of the nose.

Some spectacle frames are in the way when aiming shotgun or rifle because the stock hits the frame. The frame may prevent getting close to the sight with your eye. The Decot frame produced by Bausch and Lomb is designed so it will not be in the way when cheeking the gunstock. It is flat at the bottom so that it will not hit a closely held stock. Whether this frame is necessary for you depends upon several factors—the kind of shooting you do, your personal facial features, how you hold a gun, and the kind of comfort, safety, and good vision you want for shooting.

Optical Centers of Shooting Glasses

Since for precise aiming you want the sharpest vision you can get, it is only logical that you should sight through the optical center of

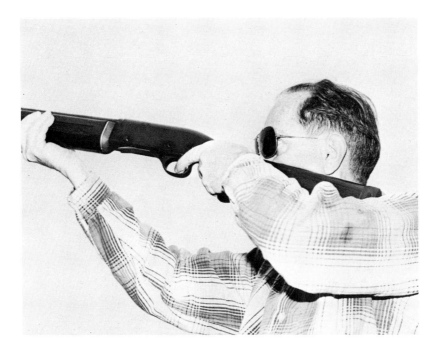

Special shooting glasses are designed so that the frame does not hit the gunstock when aiming.

a corrective spectacle lens. This is practically impossible with ordinary glasses since the optical centers are placed so that the line of sight passes through them when you are standing erect and looking at a distant object. Such a posture would be uncomfortable for most gun sighting. The only solution is to place the optical center of the lens where the line of sight enters when in normal aiming stance.

Individual sighting habits differ, as do ways of sighting different kinds of guns. Pistols are generally sighted through the upper right or left corner of a lens. Rifles depend upon the character of the gunstock, as do shotguns, but right-handers look through the upper left edge of lenses and left-handers through the upper right corners. Whether you are standing, kneeling, or prone, your eyes usually look high in the lenses.

You can easily find where the optical centers of your shooting glasses should be, provided you have the right frame size and prefer-

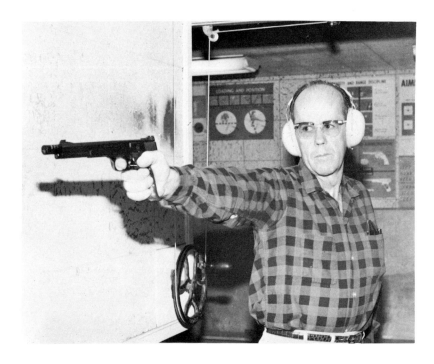

Notice how the shooter's line of sight passes through the upper right corners of his lenses. Optical centers of strong lenses may need to be placed there.

ably a lens in the frame. Cut a piece of tape about a quarter-inch in diameter. While you sight your gun with your glasses in place and properly adjusted, have someone place the tape so that it blocks off the gunsight. Take your glasses so marked when you have a new pair made in order that the optical centers may be placed correctly, particularly if you need strong lenses or if you really mean business about accurate shooting.

If you select a new frame and it has no lens on which to stick the tape, cut a piece of cardboard to insert in the frame like a lens. Punch small holes in the cardboard until by trial and error you find one right on your line of sight. Even though only one eye is sighting, the optical centers of both lenses will have to be placed in the same position; otherwise your glasses will have unwanted prismatic effects and may be unwearable.

Dominant Eye

Your aiming will be better if you sight with your dominant eye. Preferably (and usually) this will be on the same side as your dominant hand (see Chapter 3). The dominant eye is the one used in lining up two objects, gunsight and bull's-eye, for example. A complex relationship between muscles and nerves and brain determine whether or not it is on the same side as the dominant hand.

If your dominant eye is on the same side as you shoot a gun, you are fortunate. A little over 75 percent of all shooters enjoy this advantage. The shooter with crossed dominance must consider several factors such as age and experience before deciding how to proceed. If you have been shooting a long time and are no longer in your teens or twenties, stay with the side you have learned to use.

The strength of the eye dominance will also determine whether you can switch sides. It is possible to learn to sight on the same side as the dominant hand, provided the non-dominant eye has good vision. However, you may have to close the dominant eye. Practice sighting on the desired side with both eyes open; use your fingers, a paper cone, your gun and sighting technique to practice. Beginners with crossed dominance should start right off sighting on the same side as the dominant eye.

If eye dominance is too strong, it is better to give in to it and learn to hold the gun on that side. Success here too will depend upon strength of hand dominance. This is not very practical for pistol shooting since the non-dominant arm is usually less steady. A few shooters do shoot with crossed dominance, that is, right hand and left eye. When aiming a rifle or shotgun, however, two hands are on the gun to steady it and this is usually sufficient even if it is on the non-dominant side. Most people can learn to shoot this way if they are persistent. When vision dictates it, they have no choice.

With both eyes open, point one finger at a distant object. Notice which eye is used by closing one eye then the other. The one you have used in lining up your finger is the dominant eye. A more accurate way is to sight on a small distant object through a small hole cut in a piece of paper. Grasp the paper with both hands in order to get away from the influence of hand dominance. Once the object is centered in the hole, move it in to touch your face. You can easily tell which eye has been used to sight with.

Repeat the dominance test several times to be sure about it.

Generally the dominant eye is the one that has good vision, but this is not necessarily true in every case. The dominant eye may be a little more blurred than the other. However, the dominance factor is extremely important in sports involving aiming, where the dominant hand also plays a role. The dominant eye should be used if at all possible, but in cases of mixed dominance, this may not always be feasible.

If they are faulty, some of the visual skills described here can be corrected with lenses; Chapters 3 and 6 tell a good deal about this. Others can be helped by visual training and a few are not subject to change and control except indirectly, by good health care.

Visual Factors in Sighting

It is generally better to keep both eyes open when sighting. Closing one reduces the field of vision and causes the pupil of the aiming eye to dilate somewhat. This can reduce sharpness and may allow excessive light in the other eye. You can successfully keep both eyes open if you learn to ignore the image seen by the non-dominant eye. (When your eyes are directed precisely at one object, those at other distances are doubled, as described in Chapter 2.) To sight well, you must learn to ignore one image of either gunsight or target; and this takes practice.

If your eyes cannot learn to ignore the extra image when sighting a gun with both eyes, it is better to close one. Beginners should not do this but try to sight with both eyes, since they will in time learn to suppress the extra image. In shooting target, it may even be a good idea to patch off the non-dominant eye with a plastic clip over the lens on that side if it cannot be easily suppressed. Prolonged closing of one eye using the eyelid can create tension and fatigue. Hunting of course requires both eyes and they should be used in sighting. If necessary, however, close one eye only at the last minute when zeroing in on the target.

Shotgunning does not demand the precise aiming of pistol and rifle. It is more a matter of centering the gun in an area and swinging with a moving target. The dominant eye leads the way in the visual act but the broad field of view of both eyes is helpful in synchronizing body movements necessary to aim. Two eyes are better for locating the target and determining its distance and movement direction. Keep both eyes open when using a shotgun.

The type of gunsight used will greatly affect the demands upon eyesight. This subject has been discussed in some degree in Chapter 10, dealing with optical aids in the outdoors. But whatever kind of sight the hunter chooses, he must have correct distance vision for hunting or target shooting.

Sighting Rifles

A rifle is sighted by aligning the front and back sights; these may be cross hair, peep, or V-leaf systems. The front and back sights need only be centered; they need not be seen clearly. Even if the edge of each is slightly fuzzy, accurate alignment is still possible. Vision must be sharp on the target, to be certain aiming is perfect for a neck shot, for example. There is a difference in the way the various kinds of rifle sights deliver the image of the target.

Rays of light passing from the ocular surface of telescopic sights are parallel. This means the eye must be adjusted for distance seeing and need not change focus for nearer distances in aiming. This is a big advantage when the eye begins to lose its own ability to focus. Nonetheless, telescopic sights require the use of lenses which sharpen distance vision as much as possible.

Another advantage of the telescopic sight is that it magnifies the image somewhat. This can be most helpful for eyes which are incapable of sharp distance vision even with glasses, such as in cases of high astigmatism, myopia, or hyperopia, as well as with certain structural eye defects. Older eyes also tend to lose some of their sharpness and a telescopic sight may offset this. But be sure the scope has enough eye relief not to be dangerous and strike your glasses on recoil.

The least visually demanding sight after the telescopic is the open peep. The small hole of its sight also tends to make rays of light passing through it close to parallel, depending upon the peephole size and its distance from the eye. The peep does not do a perfect job, but it minimizes the need for the eye to change focus from target to sights. It increases the depth of field as does the small aperture of a camera. However, a distance correction should be worn if needed. The sights and the target cannot both be, and need not both be, perfectly clear at the same time.

The toughest sight to use visually is the iron open sight. The shooter generally wants clear vision of the distance target. When his eyes focus on it, the sights, both front and back must be slightly blurred. The human eye simply does not have enough depth of focus to encompass both target and sight on any firing piece. Using an open sight, it does not get the optical lift given in some degree by a peep and in considerable degree by a telescopic.

The open gunsights are merely centered on the target and this can be done accurately even when they are a little fuzzy. If the eye focuses for the distance of the sight, the target will become a blur, but sights can still be centered on the now fuzzy mark. Optically this is not as good a solution as if both distances were clear at once, and it presents serious problems to eyes that cannot easily change focus. Being able to see both distances clearly whether or not the eye does this adequately relates to sighting habits, pupil size, inherent depth of focus and length of the rifle, and the amount of focusing ability the eye still has. The farther the front sight from the eyes, the less focus change is necessary and the less blur is created.

Sighting Pistols

The pistol shooter has the most difficult visual task of all. The sights are generally open, though telescopic sights are made for pistols. The problems of open sights on rifles applies to pistols, and another factor which intensifies the problem even more. The pistol shooter, except when hunting, wants perfect vision of the front sight. He can tolerate no blurriness or doubt about seeing it with precision.

The pistol shooter never sees the down-range target with maximum clearness when he is aiming his pistol. It is a slightly blurred spot on which his pistol sights are centered. What he needs is the best possible vision for the distance of the front sight. This may be provided by the spectacle lens which corrects his distance vision. Or it may take a special lens correction if the shooter has reached an age when he has lost ability to focus up close.

The front sight can be sharpened by a tiny aperture in your spectacles at the position where your line of sight passes through them. Adjustable diaphragms are made for this purpose. They permit adjustment for the amount of light available in any given condition. However, they do have some limitations; the smaller the opening the sharper the focus on the front sight, yet at the same time the small opening severely reduces the amount of illumination.

The same result can be accomplished with a tiny opening in a

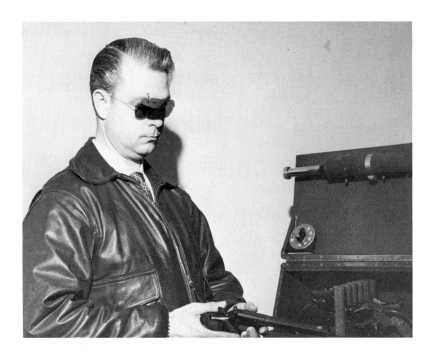

A flip-down adjustable aperture attached to glasses can be used to help sharpen front pistol sight.

piece of tape positioned in the proper location. By trial and error you can find the best size for a hole in a strip of dark tape fastened to your lens. This will aid considerably in sharpening your vision when your own focusing ability has decreased significantly; however, again it should not seriously reduce the amount of light.

Another solution to producing sharp vision for the front sight is to have a small amount of plus power (a convex lens) added to your distance prescription. Or you can simply wear a small amount of lens power for this purpose even though you require no distance prescription. Measure the exact distance in inches from your eye to the front sight of the pistol. Have the lens power made to focus for that distance.

The extra lens power need only be on the sighting eye. The other eye can wear a distance correction. This means a near lens prescription in the sighting eye and a distance lens prescription in the non-sighting eye. This can be done with a fit-over lens clipped on to the

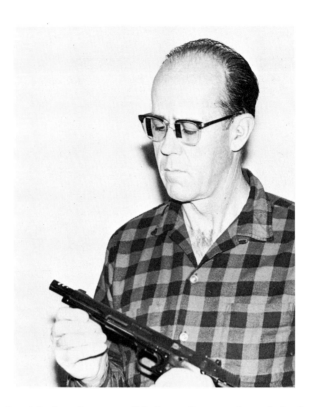

Tape on the right lens has a small hole to sharpen view of the front sight. Tape on the left blocks the eye and eliminates double vision.

side of the sighting eye when you are on the range.

Another handy solution to the problem is to wear a flip-up front frame. The frame chassis can carry a distance correction if one is needed. The flip-up front can have the small amount of lens power needed to see the front sight of the pistol. When aiming, the front is flipped down and when looking up after firing, it can be raised out of the way. In fact, the added lens power would only need be in front of the sighting eye.

Still another solution is to use a tiny bifocal in the lens of the aiming eye. This must be located exactly in the corner where your line of sight passes through the lens in firing position. This bifocal can be small and thus out of the way when you are looking and walking around the range. An ordinary fused bifocal, usually a round one, is good for this purpose.

It is also possible to cement a small wafer of plus lens on the distance correction and in this way produce needed power to see the

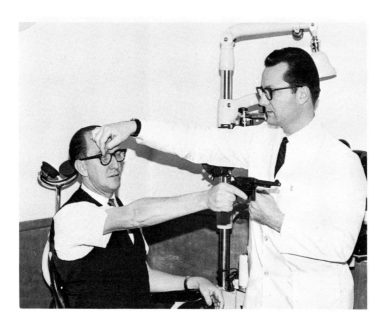

A small amount of extra lens power can be added on sighting. The best way to determine the amount is by actual testing.

front sight. This could be added on an ordinary bifocal lens. Thus, the shooter would have a bifocal in the usual downward position for near vision, a portion of the lens to look down the range, and a wafer of power in the corner of the lens (right or left as needed) to focus on the front sight. A bifocal only on one lens or the presence of an adjustable diaphragm is possible because you sight with the dominant eye, although in the case of pistol shooting, there are sometimes exceptions.

The most logical way to fire a pistol is with your dominant hand. It is steadier than the non-dominant hand and makes it easier for you to hold your body in good balance. A pistol must be sighted with the eye on the same side as the dominant hand. In most cases this is also the side of your dominant eye. The small percentage of pistol shooters with crossed dominance, meaning that the dominant eye and hand are not on the same side of the body, have no practical choice but to stick with the dominant hand.

Pistol shooters particularly must suppress the image of the non-dominant eye if they fire with both eyes open. If this is difficult, and it may well be that in firing a pistol for score, you will have to block off one eye. Closing the lid may not be easy and can build up slight tension. Certainly, it takes a bit of concentration and "effort" to keep one eye closed.

You may be more comfortable wearing a patch over your non-aiming eye. Dark plastic occluders are made which will hook onto the top of a spectacle frame. A piece of tape on your glasses covering the area in which you sight will also do the trick. For example, for the right-handed shooter the tape should be the upper right hand corner of the left lens. Thus when he turns his head to sight the pistol in a normal comfortable position, the line of sight of his left eye passes behind the patch of tape, which eliminates the double vision.

Another visual aid to aiming with comfort and accuracy is to blink and move the eyes briefly at frequent intervals to refresh the nervous system. When a person stares steadily at a fixed object, either the sight or the target, there is a tendency for his vision to blur and for small objects to disappear. This is a normal function of the eye's chemical activators.

Near-Vision Problems and Shooting

When it is no longer easy to focus your eyes for close work, shooters will find that other vision problems arise besides those of aiming a gun. Inspecting shells and the gun mechanism, even reading scores, can be difficult when eyes can no longer focus readily for near objects. When this happens, you may need lenses designed for this purpose. Your everyday glasses may do the job, but it is possible a special lens prescription will be needed.

Bifocals for hunting or use on the range should be very small and out of the way. It may be necesssary to use them for some casual near vision seeing, but if the near vision segment is large, they may interfere with walking. When the power of the bifocal is kept as weak as possible and yet is enough to deliver the focus required, ground blur will be minimized.

If you load your own cartridges or do detailed close work with equipment, it is possible you have an intense near seeing demand. This task may call for critical seeing as close as twelve to fourteen inches. Any hunter or the skeet shooter will have to see detail work if he takes his hobby indoors. Chapter 16 tells more about the sportsman's seeing problems indoors.

chapter **12**

glasses for
fishing, boating,
water sports,
and skin diving

Proper glasses will help the fisherman catch more fish. And not by using his shiny lenses as flashers on a trolling rig!

You do not believe it? Suppose any of these happened: You tie a bad knot because your eyes do not focus accurately on the monofilament line. You stumble approaching a lunker trout hole because your bifocals blur the ground. Your lure hangs up on a branch because you misjudged the distance for your cast. Many things you do when fishing depend upon vision—sizing up the terrain, selecting lures, spotting fish, casting, and moving around in all sorts of environments. Then too, some of the fun of fishing is seeing the beauty around, especially when they are not biting.

Sunglasses can be a valuable tool in the tackle box. So can corrective lenses for both distance and near vision. The reasons for wearing sunglasses, safe lenses, and good frames, covered in previous chapters, almost all apply to fishing.

About the highest brightness faced outdoors is out on the water.

Staring at the water surface is about like looking at the bright sky itself. Few eyes can, or should, do this for very long. Remember that the evidence is that excessive light on the retina of the eye for long periods of time tends to reduce the eye's sensitivity temporarily. Then too, one must prevent excessive exposure to harmful wavelengths.

Fishing

Glasses for fishing in the brilliant sun should be very dark. On medium-bright or dull days, a lens with less absorptive power is better. A sunglass particularly good for fishermen is a double gradient density lens. In addition to a medium tint, the lens has coating on the front to reflect some light. It shades from dark at both bottom and top of lens to light in the center. Result is glare reduction from sky above and water below yet permitting maximum visibility in the middle area to see around the boat, inspect tackle, or remove hooks.

Polarizing lenses have a big advantage for the fisherman. They cut surface glare and make it possible to see into the water better. That is all they do, and they cannot provide any penetrating ability beyond what is possible without glare. Such lenses are nevertheless highly advertised to fishermen as producing miracles of sight in the water; advertisers barely stop short of guaranteeing that with them you can literally guide fish onto the hook.

Reflected light is polarized by some surfaces. In simple terms, this means that all or most of the light rays are caused to vibrate only in one direction—either vertically or horizontally, for example—although the vibration could be at any angle. This light entering the eye is not useful for seeing, it merely creates a shiny image of the surface from which it is reflected. Around the water, in fishing or boating, it prevents a good view of the surface of the water and down into the water—to locate fish for example.

The sunglasses of choice for fishermen would have to be polarizing. This is also the case for other water sports—boating, or just being around the water. Water has a polarizing angle of fifty-three degrees. Polarizing lenses worn around water must be positioned at right angles to that. The problems of these lenses are that the plastic scratches, the laminated lenses may tend to separate, and the glare protection varies when the head is tilted. (The word "Polaroid" is a trade name. Polarizing lenses are sold under other names as well.)

The fisherman is the sportsman who may need bifocals the most, yet have the greatest trouble with them. Tying monofilament line is about the first activity in which he may notice that his eyes are no longer focusing up close as they used to. Tying flies, inspecting hooks and lures, even handling the line are tough visual tasks.

Optically, the solution is very simple, but practically it creates some problems. A little convex lens power in appropriate amount will relieve the eye's sagging focus. But such a lens will also blur everything more than a few feet away. This lens is perfect for close vision when snapping on a lure but no good for casting the lure in the stream.

The fisherman is in no position or mood to switch glasses in a rocking boat with a twenty-five-pound cobia circling a few yards away. He is even less ready in a rushing river tying on a new streamer during a steelhead run. The answer is a bifocal, but not just any bifocal.

Glasses made for your job probably have a large bifocal section which might interfere when fishing. The smaller the bifocal section the better for walking, or seeing the ground or a boat interior. For fishing, you need near vision only in a small area. This can be produced by a tiny bifocal, as small as fifteen to twenty millimeters.

The miniature bifocal can be positioned anywhere in the lens to suit your convenience. Located near the bottom, it permits easy look-over to get around in fishing country, while still providing plenty of near vision area. Another solution is a small bar-shaped segment set up in the lens, leaving space underneath for looking at the ground.

The fisherman must see as close as twelve to fourteen inches for detail tasks with fine line and small hook eyes, so his glasses must deliver enough power to make this possible. Few bifocals prescribed for everyday wear can do this. Whether a special prescription is needed depends upon your job and partly upon how close you want to see for fishing.

Once he is in his fifties, the fisherman who ties flies at home or works on his gear may need still a different correction. If he has a home workshop with tools arranged over a large area, he may need a lens which provides good seeing at arm's length. This could be a trifocal, or a bifocal with the top permitting clear vision out to three feet or more.

A single vision lens is good around a workbench. It can be focused for a range from eighteen to thirty inches, depending upon the wearer's eyesight. For very close work, finishing a fly or repairing a pole, a magnifier mounted on a stand works very well. Some have a light attached or you can design your own. Seeing indoors is covered more fully in Chapter 16.

Boating and Water Skiing

The boating enthusiast, whether pilot or passenger, needs the same advice as the fisherman about glasses. Good sunglasses, safety lenses, well-fitting frames are best for them both. In boats there is also a rather large risk of loss and breakage—or even a spill into the water while wearing glasses.

There are several things you can do to minimize loss of glasses around water:

1. Wear strong and tight-fitting frames which encompass the entire lens edge; be sure that the earpieces (temples) are long enough and preferably that they wrap around the ear. Special safety frames (there is a great variety of styles made for industrial uses) are built to avoid breakage and have extra deep grooves to hold the lenses in place.

2. Safety lenses should be used if there is danger of breakage in handling or from impact. They can be of heat-treated glass or of plastic. Plastic is an especially good choice.

3. The frame should have a bridge which will not injure the nose in case of an unexpected fall. A snug-fitting, all-plastic bridge would do, whereas the rocking pad might cut if it banged against the face. Even better is the special athlete's frame with a bridge of rubber padding worn in contact sports.

4. Hold your glasses in place by use of an elastic band attaching to the temples and fitting behind the head. These come with the athlete's glasses or can be purchased separately. You can easily make your own. Even a tight bathing cap will do the job, pressing the temples of the glasses against the head.

5. Glasses can be kept from sinking, in the event they do come off, by attaching some floaters to the temples. Commercial ones are available or you can make your own from strips of cork or styrofoam. Try them out in the wash basin to be sure they will hold your glasses up, then paint the floaters a bright orange or yellow so they can be easily spotted in the water.

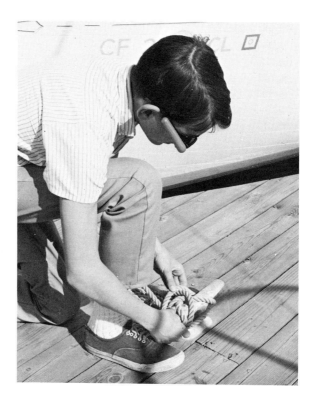

Floats attached to glasses will keep them afloat if they fall in the water.

Are glasses actually needed when water skiing? This depends upon the kind of vision you have without them. Spectacles which significantly sharpen distance seeing will add both pleasure and safety to the sport. Blurry eyesight can cause misjudgment of a wave front, even mask a floating log, or cause you to confuse the boat driver's hand signals when seen from the end of your seventy-five-foot tow rope.

You may also want to consider the role good eyesight plays in the sheer *pleasure* of water skiing. Much of the camaraderie is lost if the faces of friends are seen in a blur, and the true beauty of blue sky and sparkling water is drastically dulled by below par vision.

Once eyes begin to have trouble focusing for near objects, either reading glasses or bifocals become necessary. Without glasses, navigation charts are a hopeless blur, even instruments look fuzzy, delicate motor adjustments must be made by feel alone.

"Reading" glasses would do for charts, checking gauges, or doing fine close work but they would blur things far away, thus have to be removed. If you must also use distance correction, this would mean two pair of glasses and frequent changing from one to the other. Depending upon your seeing demands and the basic condition of your sight, bifocals may be more practical. One of the determinants is just what close work is required on the boat.

Bifocals for other jobs may be set too high or low for easy working around a boat. What is the setup of the helm? Where are the instruments? Do you stand or sit? How large are the objects you must see? Do you operate a radio, do repair jobs, run the galley, handle fishing gear, or undertake other close detail tasks? Then too, there are the purely recreational activities of reading, playing cards, even watching TV to consider.

Not only is multifocal height important, but so is the distance for which the lens is focused. Bifocals made for reading at an average sixteen-inch distance are generally too strong for an instrument panel twenty to thirty inches away. Measure how far it is from your eyes to the critical spots you must see clearly on your boat. Determine how high these areas are in relation to your eye level, standing or sitting, whichever you do. Your glasses can be made to any specification, but this requires exact measurements.

Since glare is excessive around the water, a very dark shade in sunglasses is the best protection. Only 10 to 15 percent transmission is necessary. So "ordinary" sunlenses may not be enough for long exposure to exceedingly high brilliance. Wearing a hat around the water is very helpful.

Gradient density lenses are also especially good for boating. The tint shades from dark at the top to lighter at the bottom. These lenses are sometimes difficult to wear if the gradation is too abrupt—like a tinted windshield that is dark at the top but has a sharp dividing line with the lower area. Be sure to get gradient density lenses with a smooth transition from dark to light.

Lenses with reflective coating also have value around the water. These too can be made in gradient, being highly reflective at the top and very lightly so at the bottom. But quality can vary a great deal. Examine the lens surfaces for uniformity. Only the highest quality in gradient lenses, whether tinted or reflective, are worth using at all.

What has been said about glasses around the water applies to the beach as well. Light tints are seldom satisfactory. Lying on the beach with eyes closed can lead to trouble too. It is easy to sunburn your eyelids. So wear your sunglasses when you lie back to take a nap anywhere out in the open.

Skin Diving

Skin diving has some unique seeing problems and safety itself can easily depend upon how well the diver can see. It might seem that seeing in water is somewhat hazy anyway so perfect vision is unnecessary, but this is when it is needed the most. Ordinarily it is best to wear glasses for diving if they improve visual acuity.

Light transmission depends upon the makeup of the water itself— the amount of foreign matter it contains, and this affects how well you see. In spite of diminishing intensity of light, visibility may be better at the depths than near the surface; certainly the concentration of plant life, which needs light to grow, is less there. Changes in current or tide may stir up sediment and affect visibility. Even the season cause variations; the concentration of diatoms in most areas is greatest in the spring and least in the fall.

What is happening overhead also affects visibility. Rain or wind will disturb the surface and thus scatter incident light. Underwater seeing is obviously related to outdoor brightness also. Even the angle of the sun is a factor; when it is low on the horizon, its rays are reflected from the water surface and less of them penetrate. Artificial underwater illumination is far below the brightness of sunlight. All these are factors to consider in choosing the best time to dive.

Ability to see is related to depth, regardless of water condition. The eye increases its sensitivity in dim light; this is known as dark adaptation. It is best in a healthy and rested eye but the process can be speeded up by some preadaptation.

Complete adjustment to dim light takes about an hour, although most of the useful adaptation occurs in the first few minutes. The speed of adjustment also depends upon how long the eye had previously been exposed to bright light. Thus on a sunlit beach, it would be best to wear dark glasses prior to a deep dive. They should be quite dark (physiologically, red is the best color). The necessary slow descent to adapt to pressure is helpful in giving the eyes time, but it still could be too fast for best dark adaptation.

Adaptation is needed in the other direction too. If the diver is down long enough for thorough dark adaptation, his eyes will be bothered by the bright glare when he comes up. Light adaptation is much faster; however, sunglasses may come in handy again on the beach, or in a boat, and they make it easier to see when reentering the water.

What about a tint in the diving mask plate, or in corrective glasses? Contrasts are heightened and haze cut in some degree by yellow filters and they may slightly improve seeing at depths under certain diving conditions. Thus, there may be a small advantage for a very light yellow tint in murky water or on overcast days in fresh water lakes or streams. However, all filters reduce total light somewhat. Ordinarily, the eye under water should see as "naturally" as possible with no tint in the lens and with every bit of light it can get. It is best to learn to judge colors without a tint in mask or diving glasses.

The most unusual thing about seeing under water is the distortion of size and distance. Because of the optical effects produced by water and the air lens between the eyes and diving mask faceplate, there is about a 25 percent magnification of perceived image size; this makes objects appear displaced toward the observer. Thus a fish which looks to be six feet away is actually eight, a tired diver may miss a ladder thinking it closer than it really is, and a "hundred-pound shark" may turn out to have shrunk to seventy-five pounds when put on the boat dock scale.

Practice and experience are helpful in relating the enlarged underwater image to body and limb movements which are geared to a smaller scale. It takes a lot of practice, more than most divers can get, although experienced ones arrive at a psychological adjustment and see things as a constant size both in the water and out. Judgment in spearing and reaching can be somewhat improved by keeping hands and spear in the field of view, thus everything is seen in the same, though enlarged, perspective. So the more "normal" the diver's vision is in every other respect, the fewer errors he will make in depth perception.

The underwater image distortion is also an argument for using a mask which permits as much peripheral vision as possible. This will aid overall visual orientation and minimize the water's effects. Good side vision is essential in moving around in the narrow places sometimes encountered and in spotting sea life, friendly or otherwise. Wide view masks have considerable visual advantage. Even when the diver wears a narrow-opening mask, his seeing all around can be helped by head movements. This is not hard when looking downward as the body swims along horizontally but it can be difficult when looking straight ahead. The head does not turn easily when it is tilted backwards as in swimming, and diving gear may restrict it too. Purely from a visual viewpoint, then, diving gear should not restrict easy head movement, and to look ahead and around the best, the diver should pull up and get his body vertical in the water so he can turn his head readily.

Muscle balance and all the essential visual skills are particularly important when diving because of the presence of tensions, muscular exertion, and possible anoxia. These things can upset eye-muscle balance and the result could be double vision or considerable discomfort. Even the clearness of vision is easily influenced by oxygen intake. Normal eyes are less likely to be affected, but any hazing of eyesight, seeing double, or unusual visual symptoms could be a warning to get out of the water.

Deficient color vision, however, is no real handicap for skin diving since most types of color blindness involve trouble seeing reds. This is not a common color in marine life and also red light is the first to be filtered out by water. Anyone diving to considerable depths should nevertheless be aware of any limitation he may have in color perception.

Depending upon water conditions and location, no red light penetrates beyond about 25 feet. At 150 feet orange disappears, yellow at 300 feet, blue at 400 feet, and violet at 700 feet; beyond 1000 feet light seldom reaches. Thus there is plenty of yellow, the best for visibility, in the customary diving ranges. The red-green-blind diver might have difficulty near the surface but even then he has probably learned to compensate for his faulty color perception and makes no serious errors in judgment. Keen eyesight is necessary to distinguish a lobster head from that of a moray eel, or fish from seaweed, but poor color vision probably has little to do with it.

If lens correction is necessary for diving, one solution would be to wear regular spectacles inside the mask. One difficulty is that even with flat temples (earpieces) made to fit very close to the head, some lenses must keep their position, and the mask and lens holding device which fit inside the mask to hold corrective lenses. But with insert devices to hold lenses in the mask, divers who require a strong prescription seldom obtain satisfactory vision, and there are still two tough problems left.

One of these has to do with lens placement and size. Spectacle lenses are designed to be worn a certain distance from the eye (usually thirteen millimeters) and at any other distance do not provide the desired power. In a mask, the distance would have to be calculated and the lens prescription made accordingly. At the same time, lenses must keep their position, and the mask and lens holding device have to provide the necessary stability. Lenses farther from the eye should also be bigger to provide a wide field of view, wider than for ordinary use. In the water, more eye movements are made than head movements, and this accounts for another limitation of ordinary glasses used inside the mask.

Whether corrective lenses are necessary or not, one of the big problems is fogging up of the faceplate. Certain anti-fog compounds and remedies reduce it some, but with two more surfaces of glass inside the mask, fogging is greatly increased. The temperature inside the mask is above the water temperature and this causes moisture from the breath to form on the lens surfaces. This is where the diver needing glasses really has difficulty.

There are several possible ways to solve the problem of wearing corrective lenses when skin diving. One of these is to attach an insert prescription lens inside the diving mask with metal clips or in a plastic frame in such a way as to hold the lenses in position. This is not very satisfactory since this adds two lens surfaces inside

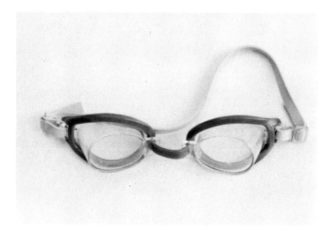

These tight-fitting goggles will keep water out of the eyes. A lens prescription can be put in them.

the mask which must be kept clean, will steam up, and reduce visibility to some degree. The lens area is small and the field of view thus reduced. Fitting and holding the lenses in position is difficult.

Some face masks are available with prescription ground in them. They correct nearsightedness only and cannot incorporate any compensation for astigmatism. The two lenses are the same power. This is a good solution for the diver with small amounts of nearsightedness, little or no astigmatism, and with the two eyes about the same.

In higher corrections, some seeing limitations are inevitable in ground faceplates. Peripheral vision becomes restricted as the power increases and the lens area becomes smaller; also the area around the prescription lens is unfinished. There is a faceplate which can be ground to individual prescription but it suffers from the same limitations.

Another method is to wear a mask that has individual eyepieces which can be replaced with prescription ground lenses. This makes

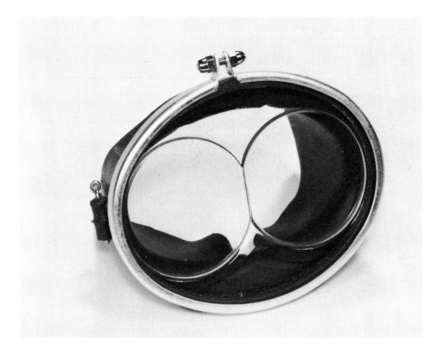

Diving mask with lenses bonded to the face plate. The large size gives a wide field. *(Courtesy of Aqua Optics)*

it possible to correct each eye individually and completely. In low-power prescriptions, such an arrangement makes a good diving mask but in higher ones some optical problems develop.

The optical centers of lenses must be placed the same distance apart as the wearer's eyes, or very close to it, or else prismatic effects are introduced. These can actually create double vision. The problem in masks is the physical one of having space to center the lenses properly. In strong powers, the decentration process creates very thick lenses on one edge or the other. If the mask has a watertight seal and the lens is ground properly on the edge, it can be well made.

One of the best methods is to bond corrective lenses to the faceplate. This can be done with any mask. Many of the mechanical problems are eliminated and the lens can be made very large. The bonding is done with Canadian balsam and holds very well with little chance of separation of the lens from the faceplate. Visibility

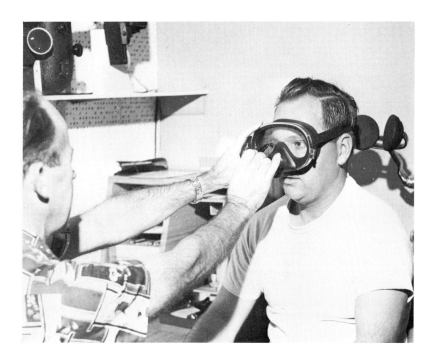

Marking a face mask for centering lenses that are to be bonded to the face plate.

and the field of view are quite good in this method even in high lens prescriptions.

Any method of fitting lenses in a face plate, or any device that positions the lens at a different distance than spectacle lenses requires careful measuring and calculations to allow for the distance. Take your mask with you so the measurements can be made.

What about skin diving for those who wear bifocals—a problem faced by most divers over age forty-five? The answer depends upon what kind of diving is done; some of it does require good near vision— to inspect any small obects held in the hand, to read a compass or watch, to examine equipment, and even to study the bottom or sunken obects. With Scuba equipment and for deep diving, bifocals may be necessary to prevent what otherwise would be blurry near vision. Bifocals can be provided by affixing lenses to the faceplate; such a device could have a lens for near use only, or both distance and near (a true bifocal) if that is necessary.

Skin divers' reactions to wearing contact lenses vary widely. Some have no difficulty while others find that the salt water creates too much irritation. Excess water in the mask can flood contacts out of the eyes. As far as visibility is concerned, they produce vision much like that of the normal eye.

chapter **13**

wearing lenses for
driving and
flying

Today's sportsman often drives or flies to fish, hunt, camp, or go on a golfing spree. Or he may drive or fly for the fun of it. Whichever the case, good vision for these activities becomes an essential part of good eyesight for sport.

It hardly needs saying that any problem with distance vision needs full correction for driving and flying—safety depends upon it. Chapter 3 tells all about visual defects and how they relate to performance; this section will deal only with those having special significance in driving and flying.

Glasses for driving and flying should be large and well fitted, as recommended for most sports. Sunglasses are essential for daytime wear and clear lenses should be worn at night. Safety lenses are recommended and for long trips or race driving, a second pair are a wise bit of insurance. The suggestions about seeing better outdoors which make up Chapter 4 will certainly benefit drivers and flyers.

Tinted Lenses and Driving

Too many drivers wear dark lenses at night. It may seem that they are beneficial because they soften the glare from headlights of oncoming cars, but, at the same time, they completely obliterate objects at the threshold of visibility, like a pedestrian at the edge of a dimly lighted street.

Some claim that yellow lenses improve night vision, but the Highway Research Board of the National Academy of Sciences reports that no color in goggles or windshields has ever been proven helpful at night. Yellow seems to be brighter and to sharpen contrasts but, like any filter, it also cuts out some light, and this is an undesirable feature in dim illumination. Yellow lenses are worn by hunters, skiers, or marksmen on dull days to help their eyes penetrate fog and haze but this is far different than night driving.

Tinted windshields reduce visibility on the road at night. If the driver is wearing tinted lenses as well, even the very light tints commonly used for regular wear, the darkening effect is compounded. One study some years ago found a higher accident rate among individuals driving under such conditions.

The trouble with tinted windshields is that in bright sunlight the tint is not enough and at night it is too much. A better windshield than one tinted uniformly is one with a tint at the top which then fades so there is no tint in the middle of the windshield and below.

Driving Glasses

Spectacle frames can actually create a seeing problem for a driver. Backing up, looking at other vehicles, and glancing "out of the corner of the eye" can be difficult if a thick frame edge is in the way. Some drivers find they have to take their glasses off to maneuver into a tight position.

Driving glasses should be larger than average for maximum visibility, but heavy, dark frame edges should be avoided. Spectacles with narrow metal rims at the sides and bottom offer the least interference to side vision. The temples or earpieces should not only be narrow, but also should be set high on the spectacle frame. Wide temples (wider than one half inch are outlawed for driving in at least one state.)

Reflections from lens surfaces are particularly annoying at night when driving or flying. A light reflective coating on the lens not only reduces the reflections but, by so doing, aids in transmitting more light.

The driver reaching the bifocal stage has some particularly annoying problems to deal with. "Reading glasses" will do for studying maps, for an occasional look at directions or a check on an

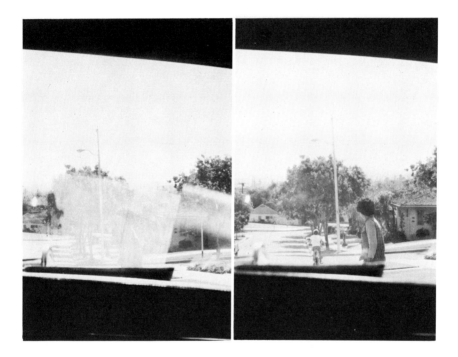

Left: The glare on the windshield is created by a map lying on the dashboard. The reflection is almost strong enough to obliterate the driver's view of a pedestrian at the curb.

Right: This photo was taken through a polarizing filter. The map reflection in the windshield is entirely gone and the pedestrian is easily visible. *(Courtesy of the Los Angeles College of Optometry)*

address, and for a glance at the instrument dials, but they blur distance vision and cannot be used at all when the car is moving. The driver who must also wear distance lenses then needs two pairs and must make frequent changes from one to the other. Bifocals are more practical.

Bifocals or trifocals made for near work jobs are usually set too high for driving. The higher the driver's seat, or the taller he is himself, the more he looks downward at the road so this means his bifocal should be positioned low in the lens. In a low car or seat, the line of sight directed at the road hits farther up in the lens and the bifocal could be higher and not interfere. For prolonged driving, bifocal position could make the difference between comfort and fatigue. Posture is a factor too; some people lean back as they drive, others hunch forward, and their preferred position determines where they look through the lenses.

Not only is bifocal height important, but so is the distance for which the lens is focused. Bifocals made for reading at the average sixteen-inch distance are generally too strong to see the dashboard clearly twenty to twenty-six inches away. This is an argument for large markings on the gauges, since the driver with bifocals would probably have to crowd forward to read small ones.

Once the eye has lost its near focusing ability, vision can be made clear at any desired near-seeing distance, but there is a limited seeing range. Bifocals made for good reading at sixteen inches, depending upon the individual's own visual condition, generally are too strong for best seeing at the twenty to twenty-six inch distance to the instrument panel.

You should measure your exact seeing distance if you want your glasses made best for your driving. Measurements from eye to dashboard and to usual near seeing areas, and the position of these areas in your line of vision, are useful information in writing a lens prescription for specific job needs. One solution is to use a bifocal which makes the dashboard visible, requiring you to read and do other close seeing jobs out a little farther than a customary reading distance. If the near seeing distance is most important, the bifocal section can be focused closer, but this will mean leaning forward a little to see the dashboard sharply.

Trifocals, incorporating a section of the lens for seeing at intermediate distances just beyond the bifocals' range, may be desirable for some drivers. The difficulty is that trifocals are placed higher than bifocals as a rule, and if they are set low, the bifocal section becomes very small, although it might be adequate. A high trifocal can interfere with distance seeing.

Seeing for Safe Driving

You can be safer on the road, at least as far as eyesight is concerned, if you remember certain things about your vision:

1. Always wear glasses if they have been prescribed for driving.
2. Do not take chances with inferior sunglasses, and never use heavily tinted lenses at dusk or at night.
3. Avoid driving if your eyes are tired, ache, or burn—be sure they are always capable of precise seeing.
4. Slow down drastically at night; in spite of how well you think you see, visibility is lowered tremendously.
5. Be sure your eyes possess *all* the vital skills for safe driving— wide fields of vision, sharp visual acuity, fine night vision, good depth perception, and perfect muscle coordination.
6. Keep your vision up to its maximum. Periodic visual analysis is the only way to be certain that eyesight is capable of making your driving as safe and pleasurable as possible.
7. If there are any limits to your visual ability, drive within those limits. Use extra rear-view mirrors, fender guides, spotlights, or special seat positions if needed.
8. Check the "visibility" of your car windows, mirrors, windshield wipers, defrosters to give your eyes every opportunity to see as safely as possible.

Glasses and Shields for Eye and Face Protection

Wearing goggles or shields for face protection is necessary in driving some sports cars and in driving motorcycles. It is risky to drive in the open air without protection. The breeze tends to dry the eyes' outer tissues and force excessive blinking. Squinting can reduce good visibility.

Protection is also needed to prevent flying objects from striking the eyes and the face. This can be anything from rock to dust. On "clean" driving surfaces, other vehicles toss up road debris in astonishing quantities, and a hefty bug can smash into the eye with plenty of force. In races and cross-country traveling, protection is even more essential.

The protective device needs to withstand tremendous impact, for example a stone coming bullet-like at a driver who is himself going sixty miles an hour. Ordinary spectacles increase the risk, even a minor blow could send splinters of glass into the eyeball. Safety lenses, plastic or glass (three-millimeter case-hardened) must be worn for eye protection.

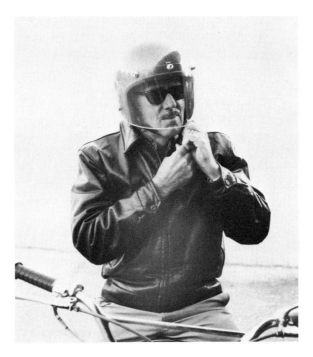

Plastic shields which are flat vertically, like this one, produce much less distortion than bubble types.

What about plastic face shields? The broad coverage they give is a great advantage. The whole face may need protection from flying debris in some kinds of sports car driving and motorcycling. In heavy dust, tight fitting face goggles are better to keep eyes clear. The two together have advantages in some circumstances.

Bubble face protectors tend to produce visual distortion. There are optical reasons for this which are independent of the quality of the plastic material. Some people are particularly sensitive to these distortions, which are produced by the small amounts of lens power created by the angle at which the line of sight passes through the curved optical surface. A sense of nausea, discomfort, headache, or fatigue can result from wearing bubble protectors, including plastic bubble goggles which fit right over the eyes. Vision can be blurry and inaccurate through the edges of any bubble device.

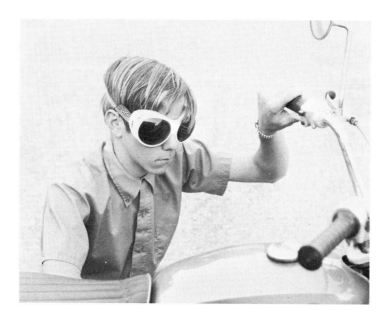

Plastic bubble lenses may be of poor quality. The wide frame edges block side vision to some degree.

Distortions in plastic shields, whether bubble or not, are less if the material is clear and homogenous. The curvature should be smooth and regular. Inspect the shield very carefully. Study its surface in reflected light. Sight on a distant object. Hold the plastic a foot away and move it slowly from side to side and up and down. Notice if the object wiggles or moves or if you can see any waves in the material itself. If so, there are imperfections of lens power.

Plastic shields which are flat vertically and curve only horizontally are much less likely to cause visual disturbance than bubble shapes. There can be small amounts of distortion in the far periphery which can be minimized by moving the head to avoid looking through the edges.

Whether the face or eye protector fits to the helmet or is worn directly on the head, its attachments should never restrict the field of view. Some goggle-type protectors worn on the face do this. Driving in traffic takes every bit of side vision you can get. Be certain that glasses, helmets, or face protectors are not blocking out anything you should see.

The soft plastic used in most face shields, some goggles, and many sunglasses scratches very easily. Be careful in cleaning. Wash off first before wiping and avoid any scratching from the grit clinging to the plastic. Replace the glasses if scratching reduces visibility at all.

Vision for Flying a Private Plane

The visual problems of flying a private plane are much the same as those of driving a car as regards corrective lenses, glare protection, and safety lenses. One goggle is designed especially for aviators, however. It is made with a front-surface reflective coating which has a clear area about the size and position of a large bifocal. This permits better visibility into the darkened cockpit without reduction in light transmission.

The day comes when pilots as well as ordinary mortals need lenses for near vision. Here are some points that the pilot must consider when describing his visual needs: At what distance from your eyes do you prepare flight plans, study maps, inspect equipment? What is the location with respect to eye level of critical near vision tasks? The average range is sixteen to twenty inches and a bifocal of ordinary size and power will do for that. But a lens producing clear vision as close as sixteen inches will probably not do in the cockpit.

What is the distance from your eyes to the instrument panel— from the closest to the farthest reading you must make? This will probably take a large bifocal which permits seeing in a range from twenty to thirty inches. Or even better might be a trifocal with a section for the instrument panel and one for some of these tasks.

Think of every prime seeing distance you have. Use a tape measure

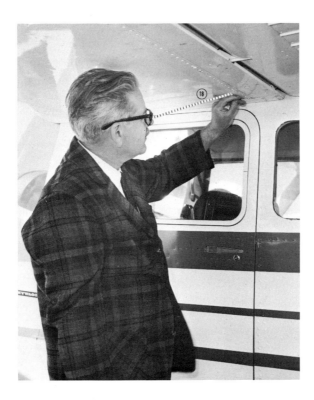

A pilot checks for water in the fuel from a distance of sixteen to nineteen inches and slightly above eye level. This kind of task may require a special lens correction. *(Courtesy of the Vision Ease Corporation)*

to actually record the exact distances from your eyes in inches. Note carefully where you must see with respect to your head position. Determine when you move your head to see, when you move only your eyes.

All of this information will be valuable in determining the size, height, and power of multifocals. Take it with you when you have your vision examined. It can be the difference between first quality visual performance and get-by seeing for you.

There is a convenient solution for the pilot to aid near vision briefly when necessary. He can wear a frame with a flip-up front. The frame itself carries the needed distance correction. The flip

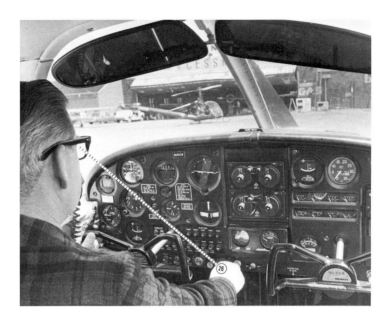

The distance from the eye to the instrument panel is about twenty-six inches; ordinary bifocals may be too strong to permit seeing at that intermediate distance. *(Courtesy of the Vision Ease Corporation)*

front (actually flipped down for use) carries a near lens power for whatever distance is needed.

If it is necessary to see overhead in the cabin, the flip-down front can have a bifocal. When flipped down, it positions the bifocal so that a small area of near vision is provided for overhead at the required distance. This arrangement can even be worn over a bifocal. Or the lens flipped down can be a bifocal in the ordinary position for downward near seeing.

Night Vision and Flying

One of the particular problems in flying, and to some extent in driving a car, is night vision. This subject was discussed in Chapter 2, but some additional points need to be made about flying.

Flying itself may reduce your ability to see at night. At high altitudes, the lack of oxygen can restrict the range of night vision. One investigator found that this change began at four thousand feet and produced a 5 percent decrease. At eight thousand feet, vision loss reached 15 percent. When this happens, the afterimages produced by lights inside the cockpit also interfere more when the pilot looks at the night sky.

How serious anoxia is for night vision depends upon individual differences and upon time. There is no way rules can be set down about altitudes or flight durations that might exceed "safe" limits. Certainly if either are considerable, a pilot who does not have a pressurized cabin should be aware that his night vision may be reduced.

It is not true that every pilot flying at seven thousand feet for several hours will suffer loss of night vision. There is not enough information to make many absolute statements about vision and flying. But it is possible that some loss of sensitivity of the eye might take place under certain conditions.

One thing the pilot definitely can do to make night vision better is to wear sunglasses during the day. This fact has been established with little doubt. A person exposed to very high brightness for a whole day may require several days spent in low illumination before his vision returns to normal. Such an impairment may be severe enough to interfere with his seeing ground lights or another plane at a distance on a dark night.

Not just any sunglasses will do. To be truly effective they must absorb at least 85 percent of the light. A neutral gray is best. If worn most of the day, and certainly during the last hours before sunset, they will improve the pilot's ability to see at night. But at night for flying he should never wear any lens tinted other than the very lightest flesh tones used in prescription lenses.

Red lenses worn just before taking off at night enhance dark adaptation. They protect the night seeing mechanism, the rods of the retina, by absorbing blue light, to which they are sensitive. Since the rate of dark adaptation is relatively slow, taking up to an hour to approach maximum, it makes sense for the pilot to start the process an hour or so before he will need maximum night vision.

Light adaptation takes place more rapidly, much of it being completed in five or ten minutes. So sitting in a "ready room" in red glasses for an hour can be a waste of time if the pilot walks down a bright corridor without the red lenses, or sits in a brightly lighted cockpit for some time before take-off. The eyes must be protected from light as long as possible if the pre-adaptation is to do any good.

Red lenses are the best, but even dark sunglasses, or simply low illumination, will help increase sensitivity to dim light. Before you go night flying, give your eyes every opportunity to adjust to the brightest conditions in which they will have to operate. Keep instrument lights and cabin illumination as low as is consistent with other seeing requirements.

Once in the air, you can do several things to preserve your light sensitivity. Avoid using any more light inside than necessary. Shield light sources so there are no glare spots. Each time you look at a bright source, dark adaptation drops rapidly, and it takes three or four times that long to get back full night vision. Keep your eyes moving too in order to prevent washing out certain parts of your retina, especially the central area.

Since the night vision mechanism is sensitive to blue light, that color should not be used for illumination inside the cockpit. Red is better; in red light the pilot can see what he needs and still protect

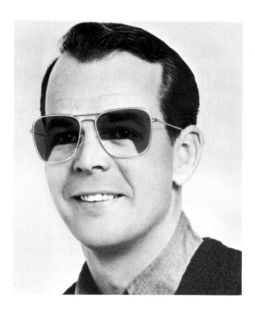

Pilot's glasses: the front surface is coated, with the bottom left clear for seeing inside the dark cockpit. (*Courtesy of Bausch & Lomb*)

the sensitive visual cells of his retina. Of course, much depends on the kind of flying. Over a huge city so much light reaches the eyes that they do not need maximum dark adaptation—in fact they could never reach it. But hunting for a tiny landing strip in remote country takes all the night vision possible.

Since the night seeing system of the eyes is quite sensitive to blue, that is a good color for marker lights. They can be spotted at great distances, especially in blackout conditions. Once down on the ground where overall brightness, even at night, may call some of the day seeing mechanism into action, red and green are readily visible and have value in signaling.

Some pilots who have perfectly clear vision in the daytime develop a definite blur in their vision at night. This is known as night myopia (nearsightedness). It happens because the light is dim and is not unique with flying. The dim light causes the pupil of the eye to enlarge and expose the edges of the optical system in such a way as to change its total refractive power. The result in some eyes is to throw distant images out of focus.

If you have blur at night, whether flying, driving, or just walking, you may find that squinting sharpens your vision some. If so, the problem can probably be corrected with lenses. (Yes, it is sometimes necessary to have a different lens prescription for night than for daytime!) Tell your optometrist if you fly at night or have special problems seeing in dim light. Have him test your eyes under low levels of illumination to determine if you might have night myopia.

Some blur at night occurs because the eye has nothing to look at. In fact, a similar condition arises in the daytime at high altitude and is called space myopia. When the pilot looks out of the cockpit, the eye is in a dilemma with nothing to focus on; even faint lights are at an indefinite distance. Under such circumstances the eye tends to adjust to a middle distance, making far away objects blurry.

There is no way to correct space myopia with lenses because it is variable. Once the eye locates something to focus on, it does so and the myopia is gone. However, its effects can be minimized by keeping the eyes moving. Look from cabin to ground to wing tips; avoid simply staring into space and allowing the vision to degenerate into a blur.

Moving eyes around is a good practice in night flying. It helps to locate planes in the air or to pick up ground clues the pilot is searching for. The eye tends to adapt and lose sensitivity to what it is looking at. Especially at night, some of the peripheral visual field is more sensitive than central vision. So sweeping the eyes around puts this radar screen to work over a large area.

No matter how good one's eyes, seeing to fly at night is more difficult for purely physical reasons. Objects are harder to see because they are dimmer. On this basis alone, they look farther away than they really are. It is also hard to judge their speed, position, and identity. If glasses are needed at all for distance vision, they are even more important at night.

Visual Illusions and Flying

A number of illusions occur in flying which are unique to this activity. One can have sensations of the plane banking or changing altitude when actually it is flying perfectly level. The horizon can appear in the wrong place, stationary lights can seem to move, and images can fade away.

There things happen because the human senses are not highly reliable in determining orientation in space. The sense of touch (tactile sense, as from the pull of gravity), the sense of balance (as controlled by the vestibular mechanism in the inner ear), and vision all have something to do with determining where one is in space. But these senses can all be fooled—and very easily under certain flying conditions.

"Seat of the pants" flying is not at all accurate. The pull of gravity cannot be relied on to tell what the plane is doing—for example, if acceleration is gradual and sound of motors not noticed, increased speed does not register. Tilts as much as ten to twenty-five degrees cannot be detected by blindfolded subjects. Reversal effects occur after steep banks in one direction. So the sense of equilibrium cannot be trusted to provide more than gross information.

Vision provides the majority and the most reliable clues to spatial orientation. One of the remarkable functions of the eye is that of constantly reporting information about where the body is with respect to its environment. But if it interprets the surroundings incorrectly, the body's orientation will be totally wrong. For example, you cannot tell if you are upside down from sight alone if your whole visual field is also upside down.

Many experts in aviation who have studied disorientation extensively recommend that pilots rely on instruments and ignore their bodily and visual sensations no matter how strong. Barring mechanical defects, instruments are more trustworthy since they are not subject to illusions.

Peripheral vision is helpful in maintaining aircraft roll attitude in clear weather. In fact, it is so hard to ignore, that one tends to become dependent upon it. But when shifting to instrument flight, central vision is the most important. The pilot should be able to shift from one to the other very quickly. To do this effectively he must keep both central and peripheral visual systems alert as much as he can. So maintain awareness of "seeing things out of the corner of your eye." When looking at the whole field of space, sky, and ground below, pick out objects to look at now and then to keep your central vision active. When flying on instruments, keep side vision busy noticing the interior of the cabin.

The eye tends to adapt to a fixed set of conditions. Indeed, certain kinds of images disappear when they are experimentally stabilized on the retina. The visual system is built to detect *changes* in the world about it. So try not to stare into space, or "freeze" on the horizon or a cloud formation. Even if there is nothing to see out the windshield, glance around the cabin, look outside, check the instruments, keep eyes busy with different images. No need to stare constantly at the instruments. When there is no ground or discernible sky pattern visible, the flyer is a good candidate for disorientation.

It is best not to trust your judgment of lights, especially single lights, until they have been verified beyond a doubt. Check instruments also to be sure visual images make sense according to what they indicate. Be especially careful when the ground cues are unfamiliar.

A sort of mystic sensation can occur when there is nothing to orient with—as when surrounded by fog. This is not so much faulty orientation as an inability to achieve any sort of localization at all. Total blackness gives the same feeling although it is not quite as confining. In either case, the pilot has no choice but to fly blind and rely on instruments. But problems arise when he tries to shift quickly back to visual contact. For many minutes, maybe even a few hours, he has had no visual frame of reference for orientation other than a formless field ahead. It may take him some time to adjust to judging by eyesight again. Objects first coming into view may seem unreal or be located incorrectly.

Avoid white-out effects by not peering too hard into space. Vary attention. Moving the head and body somewhat can reduce the effects of misreading what the visual sense reports. You can keep your visual perception sharp and alert, rather than lulled to dull-ness, but remember that vision cannot always be trusted. Learn when illusions are most likely to occur when flying. Keep peripheral vision alert, avoid staring, and move the eyes frequently and rapidly. Then above all, be sure to check instruments even though there is also visual contact. Be sure they work perfectly so you can really trust them.

These last suggestions are good whether in plane, boat, or auto-mobile. And by working for improved perception, as described in Chapter 4, you should enjoy vision that is better and safer for oper-ating any kind of vehicle.

chapter **14**

some special

visual problems

in sports

Skiing

One of the biggest of all seeing problems for the skier, or anyone in the snow, is glare. The professional, or the person who is outdoors a great deal, has less of a problem, since his eyes are accustomed to the extreme brightness of sun or snow, but many of America's skiers are indoor workers. They spend a good part of their lives in artificial light whose maximum brightness is a thousand times less than that encountered on ski run. Goggles and other forms of eye protection aid by keeping wind, or snow or sleet, from interfering with vision, and this is reason enough for using them. But glare reduction is an even more important value.

Long exposure to glare can produce "snow blindness." This comes from a swelling and irritation of the outer tissue of the cornea (the clear front covering the eye). It takes long exposure, however, and is not likely to occur under ordinary skiing conditions.

It is caused by ultraviolet light. This is significant in skiing because although the percentage of ultraviolet in sunlight at sea level is only 1 to 2 percent, at higher elevations it is 5 to 6 percent.

It might seem that a cap would eliminate the difficulty if its bill cut the overhead glare. But most of the ultraviolet rays entering the eye are reflected from the snow and reaches two to four times the intensity of direct sunlight. In fact the sun need not be out at all to produce glare. Even on an overcast day, there may be as much ultraviolet in light reflected from the snow as in direct sunlight itself.

What lens tint should you use? No single shade will meet all the conditions the skier must face. With a bright sun after a snowfall, you would need a dark filter to do the job, but this would cut out too much light on dull days. Those who ski a great deal usually own several pairs in different tints. Another solution is the type of goggle which permits changing the plastic filters so that one of the proper density can be inserted in position in the eyepieces.

Color is important. Darkness alone is not enough. The deeper the tint the more light is filtered out, and within limits this is desirable. But more significant is whether or not the lens filters out ultraviolet. You cannot tell this just by looking at the lens; however, a purple, or blue, or violet lens is more likely to transmit ultraviolet than a color at the other end of the spectrum—a green, yellow, or red (red is not recommended).

Opposite the ultraviolet in the visible spectrum is infrared and good filters also block much of it. Usually the best filters are in the middle range of hues visible to the human eye: green, yellow-green, amber, light brown and gray. Neutral grey would have to top the list of recommended tints for wear in sunlit snow.

Many skiers find that certain shades of orange and yellow enhance shadow contrast in flat lighting and on gray days, making it easier to pick out the contours of the moguls. But for the very bright days few ski goggles absorb as much light as they should. Use a very dark plastic insert for the bright sun.

The average amateur's participation in winter sports is so brief that the glare protection he uses need not be scientifically perfect. Plastic lenses will not injure sight nor create serious seeing hazards for limited usage. But the professional, or serious amateur skier who undergoes any long exposure to sun in winter should have the best available lenses with ideal transmission quality and the ability to absorb both infrared and ultraviolet rays.

Unfortunately, few lenses in ski goggles are scientifically compounded to filter out ultraviolet. A survey of a number of them failed to produce information on their exact wavelength filtering properties. However, plastic naturally does a pretty good job of blocking ultraviolet. Tints are added to glass to be most effective in absorbing it. For long exposure at high altitude, you should be sure that whatever eye protection you wear absorbs ultraviolet.

Filtering out infrared is something else. Plastic will not hold a stable dye which will absorb infrared; glass does a better job. It is not known whether long wavelengths have long-range effects on eye health—some think perhaps they do. This risk is probably not worth worrying about to the skier who spends but a few days outdoors on snow each year, but for the professional it might be.

Most ski goggles have plastic lenses. Flat lenses are best. Sharply curved plastic goggles, especially bubble shapes, can be full of distortions. Unless they are especially well made, curved ones are not as good as flat or those curved in only one meridian. The quality of the plastic is significant, as is the kind of light it absorbs and the stability of the tint.

Good quality ski goggles with scientifically compounded tints for use around the snow are now being produced. Most of these lenses are made in Europe and are plastic. The tints come in a variety of colors to meet various brightness conditions and a selection of shapes and styles are available for various types of goggles.

Face-form spectacles can be made in prescription and in any desired tint. The typical ski goggles are a device which fits to head and face with a soft padding of rubber or fur; most of them have plastic protective shields which cannot incorporate a lens prescription. However, certain styles are designed with slots at the sides to permit wearing of eyeglasses under the ski goggle.

Thus there is no reason for people who wear glasses to be dubious about skiing. Their vision may be more adequate than many without glasses who need them and do not know it. Proper use of tints and safety goggles can make seeing and skiing perfectly safe for the person who must wear glasses.

Bifocals are not generally usable for skiing since they would make the ground look blurred up to ten or fifteen feet in front of you. This is a distance within which you must often focus your attention, so you will want a distance prescription only for this sport.

Glasses and goggles are a nuisance in certain kinds of weather because they fog or ice up. Everything from hot air injection on

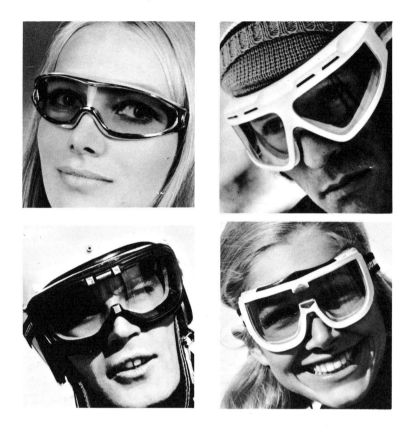

Ski goggles are available in a large variety. They should fit snugly and provide a broad field of view. *(Courtesy of the Garcia Ski Corp.)*

the lenses to windshield wipers has been tried with little practical success. Many experienced skiers use two pairs of goggles, keeping one inside the jacket, next to the body, where they will dry out. One way to minimize the problem is to wear glasses with plastic lenses; these can be made in prescription. Another aid is to have lens surfaces well ventilated, even if this means cutting extra holes in the rubber frame. And of course a good supply of dry handkerchiefs or paper napkins can be valuable. To use them you may have to stop in the middle of your best run, but continuing in your iced-up state can easily bring you—or another hapless skier—to grief.

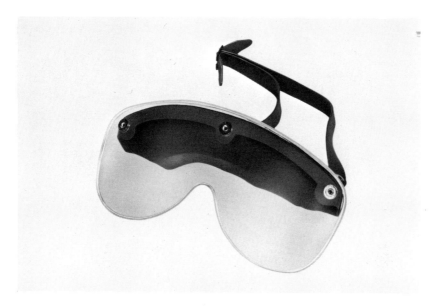

This ski shield can be worn over other glasses; it has interchangeable lenses in several tints. *(Courtesy of Bausch & Lomb)*

It is possible to make a fog resistant lens by a combination of two plastic lenses with an air space. This permits the front lens to be cold and the inside one warmer without the air which touches the surfaces reaching the dew point. This is a specially made lens which offers a good solution to the fogging problem.

Contact lenses are an ideal way to eliminate spectacles but do not provide a total solution for skiing. Contact lens wearers are generally more light sensitive than average, so with snow glare a more intense problem, sunglasses become especially necessary and may be needed in dark tints to make contacts truly comfortable. Wind protection is also needed, so ski goggles are generally worn even with contact lenses. Do not get contacts for skiing alone. If you wear them for other reasons, you can probably ski with them, but make provision for adequate glare protection besides.

What has been said about skiing is the same for any outdoor snow sports—ice skating, snowmobiling, or just plain being out in the snow. Glare protection is advisable, especially for long exposure.

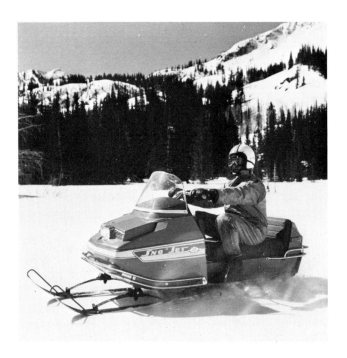

Good glare protection as well as head and face protection is provided by a helmet and goggles for snowmobiling. *(Courtesy of Sno-Jet Inc., Quebec, Canada)*

Mountain Climbing

Altitude increases the amount of ultraviolet exposure, as was pointed out earlier. Consequently, sunburns are likely at high altitudes and climbers find it advisable to protect the face, not only to avoid the cold but also to prevent serious burn.

Even when a climber is not on snowfields, once he gets above timberline, he can encounter strong glare from rock unbroken by foliage. Inexperienced climbers are often fooled by cloudy days when the light does not seem very bright. Light tints in lenses can be used here to add to visual comfort. On snowfields, dark tinted, close-fitting "glacier goggles" are usually worn to insure that the eyes are protected from all sides.

Seeing problems at high altitudes may be brought on by lack of oxygen. The retina is very sensitive to the amount of oxygen available, and if there is not enough the result can be blurry or even double vision, depending upon the person's basic visual condition. For this reason, any error of refraction of the eyes or muscle imbalance should probably be corrected (by wearing lenses if needed) for mountain climbing, even though the demands on vision itself are relatively mild.

Hiking, Rowing, Canoeing

Sunglasses are desirable whenever prevailing conditions involve considerable bright light. Generally, around the water you will be more comfortable with tinted lenses. For hiking in the woods, you probably do not need them.

But should corrective lenses be worn for outdoor sports such as canoeing or hiking? The answer depends upon what the correction is for and how strong it is. Not wearing glasses during physical exertion will not change eyesight. Lenses make one see better and provide comfort, but outside of a few instances in which they are prescribed for young children, they do not correct the condition itself.

During many strenuous outdoor activities, visual acuity, depth perception, and speed of recognition need not be at peak performance. On the other hand, the lens correction will enable vision to function most easily. There is no reason glasses cannot be worn if they fit well, stay on, and are not too hot. An elastic band attached to the temples and fitting behind the head will keep them in place. Plastic lenses in a very light frame will keep the weight down and provide maximum comfort.

Archery

Experienced marksmen aim with both eyes open. This is the best method even when the archer uses a sight mounted on the bow or ground markers in front of the target. Sighting is done with the dominant eye since the non-dominant eye can more easily suppress its registering of the doubled image. If the tip of the arrow is fixated, the target or marker is seen double; while if the distant object is fixated, the arrow tip is doubled. It is better to keep both eyes open and to learn to ignore the doubled image than to uncomfortably close one eye.

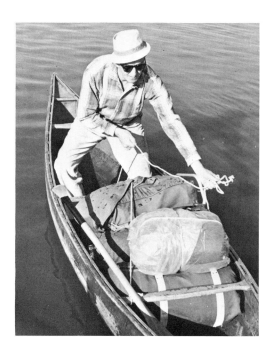

Glasses for active jobs may need to be held on with an athletic band behind the head.

Bowsights operate much on the same principle as gunsights (Chapter 11). The premium is on distance vision when sighting. If the sight blurs, then a lens designed to focus for the distance of the sight would be helpful.

Hitting a moving target in bowhunting takes fast and precise judgment of speed and distance. Anything that interferes with your eyes working smoothly together can cut down effective seeing. Depth perception also is important in hunting and in range shooting. You must estimate distance, height, and angle with pinpoint accuracy to make a good score. It never hurts to test your judgment now and then, and to practice improving it. Measure your average step. Get out on the range, judge the distance to selected points, and step them off to see how accurate you are.

Older archers may wear bifocals for ordinary seeing and some lenses can create problems in archery shooting. Normal sighting is done through the top of spectacle lenses, thus bifocals are not likely to interfere. However, if the spectacles were made with a higher-than-average bifocal, a trifocal, or with a prescription for a particular working distance, they would not be good for archery.

Some close vision is used to inspect arrow shafts for cracks, splinters, and alignment; check the feathering; examine the arrowhead for imperfections, and, upon occasion, to identify arrow characteristics by a personal numbering system. This requires good near vision and may call for bifocals for the archer who has passed his mid-forties. These near vision needs are all well downward, and a bifocal should be set very low so as not to interfere with sighting downward towards a ground marker or for walking over rough terrain.

Bowhunters run some risk of lens breakage in traversing rough country. Safety lenses are the best bet to prevent an accident which might ruin the hunt, and to protect eyes from injury from a sharp twig or a speck of dirt.

The best choice for any archer regardless of age, is a special pair of glasses with a full distance correction, made in a large-sized well-fitted frame and tinted to suit conditions in which he shoots.

Golf

Of all the general visual skills so valuable outdoors, as described in Chapter 2, depth perception is one of the most important for golfing. Visual estimate of distance from ball to pin directs muscles to hit the ball with the right amount of power.

The golfer should become an expert in judging distance. One way is to practice. Estimate a distance, then step it off. Keep at it until accuracy is high. Another way is to use a range finder, but for practice only. Small devices easily carried in the pocket can be used to determine exact distances, but they are illegal for actual play under U.S.G.A. rules.

If you wear glasses designed for use at home or for work, they may be all wrong for golf. Indeed, because of the special demands golf places on distance seeing, it is possible you may require a special prescription. Glasses made for other purposes or for "general wear," may of course be suitable for golf. Many are. But you should have yours checked out to be sure.

When you have your vision examined, explain exactly how you use your eyes while playing. Do you tilt your head and use your left eye in sighting on the ball during your back swing? How closely do you study the grain of a green? Does glare bother you? Are you constantly over- or underjudging distances? Can you easily read the score and inspect the ball? How far away do you hold them to see? Once your optometrist recovers from the shock of getting so much good information, he will write a better prescription for your needs than ever before.

When a golfer is in his mid-forties to early fifties he may have to face the bifocal question. For many, there is no great problem since the near vision demands for golf are rather mild. They do exist, however, and need solving for some people.

A pair of reading glasses can be put on to check the score card, examine the ball, or even to study the green but doing this is a nuisance. Especially if a distance correction is necessary, a bifocal is the best solution. For golf the bifocal segment should not be set high in the lens. If it is, it can blur the ball when the golfer is using the longer clubs. Trying to look over the bifocal segment results in an unnatural head tilt that throws the body out of balance. Ordinary bifocals are also generally too strong for casual near seeing needs on the course.

Special bifocals were designed for golfers years ago. They have a tiny, round segment set very low in the lens. This can even be positioned off to one side, depending upon whether the player is right- or left-handed, to get it out of his way when he is addressing the ball. This lens provides an adequate near vision area. Other types of bifocals can be used but they should be set low in the lens.

Site and location of the bifocal are not the only considerations. Its power should not be too great. A lens prescription for close work and prolonged reading would ordinarily create considerable blur for any point more than eighteen to twenty inches away. The golfer's bifocal should be as weak as possible, focused just close enough to see the scorecard, leaving as much outward range as possible to look at the green and minimize blur on the ground. Be certain that these factors are considered when your prescription is written.

Trifocals are generally out of the question on the golf course. So are many other special multifocals which interfere with distance vision, walking, or looking at the ball to drive, chip, or putt. Just as each club is designed for a certain purpose, so are glasses tailored to exact vocational or recreational needs—and this is particularly true of multifocal lenses.

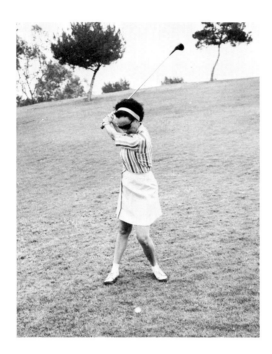

An ordinary bifocal set high in the lens can interfere with a shot like this, making it necessary to duck the head more than is natural.

Camping

Why put camping down as an outdoor activity that may require glasses? The activities involved in camping rarely place any tough demands on eyesight. But good vision provides the fullest enjoyment of natural beauty—the sky, the forest, a stream, a mountain, the desert. Camping is in many respects a visual experience, and for any visual experience you want your seeing to be at its best. So keep your seeing needs in mind when you run through your checklist of equipment. If lens corrections or sunglasses will make a substantial difference to you, take them along.

good vision
can improve
photography

Cameras are a part of outdoor life. Beauty and memories captured on film are often among the sportsman's prized possessions. Yet most people know very little about the visual performance necessary for photography. Two major aspects should be noted. One is seeing properly and the other is making the best picture of what is seen.

Many photographers, both professional and amateur, are uncertain if their vision is what it should be for camera work. Anyone using a camera frequently should first of all determine if he possesses the visual skills described in Chapter 2.

Bespectacled photographers especially have plenty of seeing problems. Frames and lenses get in the way when they are looking through viewfinders and the picture composition suffers. Lens prescriptions are seldom designed for the photographer's very specialized seeing needs either. To get the proper lenses he must know exactly what these needs are for the kind of camera work he does.

To produce a truly good picture, you should be able to see every detail of figure and ground. This means visual acuity should be the best it is possible to get. But it takes a lot more than sharp sight to create an unending series of "ohs" and "ahs" photos.

If you are nearsighted, or have much astigmatism, your distance vision will be blurred and should be corrected. Astigmatism particularly can make things look distorted and as a result pictures may never turn out as expected. It is possible to compensate momentarily by squinting the eyelids down (like getting better focus with a narrow aperture stop), but of course glasses do a better job.

Even the farsighted eye can create a special problem in photography. Fatigue and eyestrain can occur from its use, especially in order to see up close. Strain is bad enough but even worse are the inaccuracies farsightedness can cause when the photographer is localizing the central figure, scanning a scene hurriedly to get a candid shot, and especially when he is looking back and forth between far and near objects.

The focusing mechanism of the photographer's eye should operate with maximum dexterity. This goes for all eyes, whether nearsighted or farsighted. There is a special skill involved in aiming the eyes and focusing them for a number of points in the whole scene while the action is going on, the subject is fidgeting, or clouds are rushing to block the sun. "Don't hurry" is sound photographic advice, but sometimes there is no choice.

Blurred vision can be an asset—up to a point. Sometimes balancing the picture and deciding on the major aspects of its composition can be easier without the distraction of minute detail. The person with mildly blurred sight could take his glasses off at this stage. Or focus can be relaxed (easily done by the farsighted eye), to soften the sharp detail as the picture is composed. Even squinting the lids way down can create the same effect.

Judging Amount of Light

Be careful to avoid errors in judgment when light conditions change suddenly. Remember it takes five minutes or more for your eyes to adjust well to increased brightness. Since dark adaptation is much slower, allow fifteen to thirty minutes for your eyes to get used to darkroom lighting or that of any very dim environment.

No matter how experienced the photographer, he can be deceived about correct exposure time when a sudden change in cloud cover occurs, or when the subject moves into shade. Exposure is especially difficult to judge while the eye is adapting to new light levels. Take time to evaluate a scene when lighting conditions have changed. Rely on light meters and photometers for accurate findings, because your eyes are not reliable for quantitative measurements. However, use your eyes to judge contrasts and to determine the lighting you will need for artistic effects; for this they are better than any mechanical device.

Experience and judgment are necessary to modify what the light meter says. Assuming it is working properly, the meter reads the amount of light correctly. But it may be gathering most of its information from the sky, while the subject of the photo is in open shade. Several light meter readings in different directions should be taken. But the eye itself in such a case can help decide which to use.

Sunglasses of any tint can affect your judgment of brightness and result in overexposure, since you will think it less bright than it really is. Learn to judge brightness the same way each time you take a photograph, either with or without your sunglasses. If you have just put sunglasses on or removed them, allow time for adjustment before you trust your judgment of light conditions. Remember that if you have just taken tinted lenses off the light will appear stronger than it really is, so you may tend to underexpose your film.

Depth Effects

Many of your pictures will be better if you can accurately judge depth and distance. A split-field range finder can eliminate a lot of guesswork, but it takes visual evaluation to decide what should, or should not, be in good focus along with the central subject. Practice making some estimates of distance, then check them with your range finder. Learn to use shadow, size, color, overlap, and perspective to aid depth discrimination.

Depth perception is enhanced to some degree by the two eyes, though this factor is exaggerated in the example of stereo testing devices. In stereophotography three-dimensional or 3-D, effects are obtained by taking two photos from slightly disparate positions, then imaging one on one eye and one on the other. The eyes receive slightly different images because of their lateral separation of about two and a half inches, and this difference creates a depth effect. A stereo picture can be enhanced by taking the two photos with a wider separation.

Normal two-dimensional photos can never simulate the exaggerated depth of a stereo creation, but the huge majority of photos produced on a flat surface still appear to have depth in some degree. This is so because they possess some of the other qualities which create the depth effect. The photographer should learn to take fullest advantage of them.

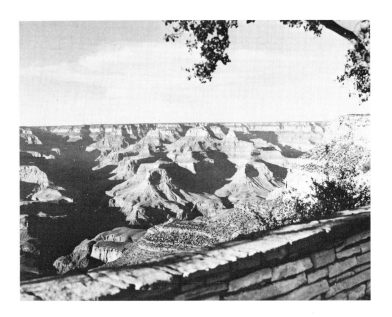

Foreground objects, the stone wall and tree branch, and the long shadows create lots of depth in this picture.

To visualize how a scene would look when on a flat surface, close one eye, thus minimizing the 3-D effect. The difference may not appear great but will help in composing and evaluating a scene. The viewer is forced to rely on the depth factors that influence one eye alone—such elements as shadow, overlap, line convergence, brightness, and, of course, color.

Shadow adds a great deal to the depth effect. That is why experts advise against using flat lighting. For example, the Grand Canyon photographs much better in early or midmorning and midafternoon to late evenings, when strong shadows make the formations stand out. So not only photograph when the light creates shadows, compose in such a way as to enhance the shadow-created depth in the picture.

Move the subject to take advantage of shadows, or change your position to make the most of them. Wait until there are long shadows or create them by flash or floodlights—depending upon the effect you want.

Depth can be added by changing viewing position so that one object overlaps another. If it does overlap, it is obviously in front of another, and this emphasizes the depth. All that may be needed is to shift a vantage point to improve the photo. Or if objects can be arranged in the scene, place the one you wish to appear in front of the other.

The same result is achieved by using a foreground object. Especially on shots involving long distances, adding something in the foreground—a person, an overhanging limb, etc.—creates more depth. Objects in a picture can be arranged to accomplish this or camera position or angle can be selected to include a foreground object.

It is essential to remember that the shrunken size of the photo also reduces distance. The beginning photographer stands at a vista in the Great Smokies, grabs his camera to record forever the magnificent view of mountains disappearing in the distance, then finds that on a wallet-sized print the whole scene is disappointingly flat.

The print never has going for it all the clues the eye can use right on the spot. Color is one of the factors. Black and white prints must have shadow, overlap, distance parallax and proper use of brightness to increase depth. With color, they are less imporant but not unimportant.

Convergence of lines also creates a depth effect. Shooting straight down a highway increases the illusion of distance more than if the picture is taken across prairie land. Take advantage of this principle by designing a set with converging lines or composing to get most of the effect.

Brightness also influences the depth effect. Bright objects appear near, dim ones far. If there is any way to control brightness of objects in the picture, add depth by placing dim ones in the background. In the studio, heighten the front lighting, reduce the back light.

Improving Composition

A fundamental principle of visual perception is the law of good form. This says the human visual mechanism tends to see things in an orderly manner, in good balance, in *good form*. By the same token, then, it judges visual images as being "good" if they have balance and symmetry. Compose pictures with this in mind.

Nature tends to have a great deal of symmetry and balance. But a picture captures only a small segment, and this could be very bad form. The angle at which a picture is taken can destroy balance. So can cutting an object in half—even though there may be no choice, since slicing several objects in pieces may be necessary to get the central figure in the frame.

Don't make a photo top-heavy by having a huge object on one side, nothing to balance it on the other. Good form means balance, regularity, orderliness, and smooth flow. Compositions that have these qualities are "good," in one sense of the word.

Watch the edges of the viewfinder very carefully. There is no cropping on a color transparency, though with black and white it may be possible to enlarge out some errors. A slight change in aiming direction, moving closer to or farther from the subject, can eliminate unwanted material in the photo. Some material may be "unwanted" because of what it is or where it is, or because it may destroy the picture's good form.

Special effects occur when the fundamental laws of perception are violated. Disorderliness can make an artistic picture. Yet strangely enough, to be good, there has to be some orderliness to the disorder. Violating the principle of good form has to be done with discipline— distortions that completely upset the total balance of a piece of art generally appeal to very few.

If the photographer upsets the law of good form by accident, he is lucky if he gets a good picture. By design he may create an unstable pattern that results in some exotic effects. These are typified by various op art patterns. Though not appearing in nature, they do illustrate by exception the role of balance and symmetry so important to the kind of pleasant photograph the outdoorsman wants to produce.

The foregoing is not meant to be even remotely a lesson in art. It has only pointed out some of the rules of perceiving that can be helpful to the photographer. They can be put to work very easily whenever he looks through his camera. These are suggestions that will make pictures better for those who love to photograph the outdoors. But how successfully they work partly depends upon how effectively the photographer can see through his viewfinder.

Eye-Level Viewfinders

The viewfinders found on single-lens reflex cameras, instamatics, movie cameras (except open viewers held right to the eye) are opti-

cally similar as far as the eye is concerned. The light rays leaving the
back surface of the finder lens are parallel. This is the same as light
from optical infinity. Therefore, spectacles which correct distance vision
should be worn when focusing such systems.

It makes no difference whether the viewfinder utilizes a split-
field, ground-glass, or a Fresnel lens—to use it effectively sharp vision
is essential. Use the eye with better vision if your eyes are not equal.
Or use the dominant eye, which is usually the sharpest as well (see
Chapter 2).

A few cameras have an eyepiece which can be adjusted for small
errors of refraction. This serves to correct regular conditions, nearsightedness or farsightedness, but it cannot compensate for astigmatism. Thus the adjustable eyepiece produces good vision for only
a few people. For them, the advantage is great since their eye can
be crowded close to the viewfinder without interference of glasses.

Viewfinders are generally made so that the entire field is visible
only if the center of the system's exit pupil falls at the center of the
entrance pupil of the eye. However, spectacles are designed to be
positioned about half an inch in front of the cornea, and they may
prevent the eye from getting in the right position. The result can

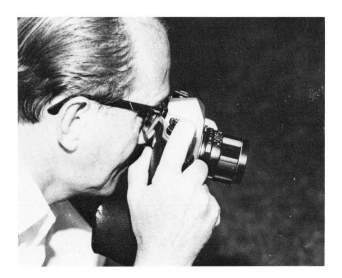

With glasses it is nearly impossible to get close enough to the view finder
to see the full frame; yet corrective lenses are necessary for sharp focusing.

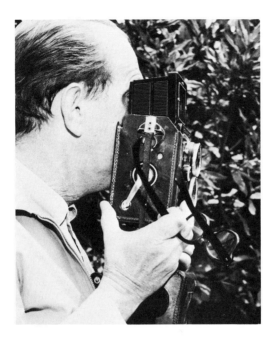

Focus with glasses on; take them off and crowd close to frame the picture, unless vision is too badly blurred without them.

be loss of a part of the picture when composing and framing. For black and white photos that can be enlarged and cropped, the problem is not so serious, but on color film and slides unwanted objects may be visible on the finished product.

Depending upon the intensity of your visual problem and how blurred you are without glasses, one solution is to remove your lenses when framing so you can crowd close to the view finder. Leave them on for focusing when you must see sharply. Taking your glasses off for every shot is a nuisance but it can improve your product. If you do this, attach your glasses to a cord or chain around your neck so that when you take them off you avoid holding or dropping them.

A partial solution is to have your lenses fitted as close as possible to your eyes. It may be necessary to modify the power for the different eye-to-lens distance. Select a frame that can be adjusted close to the eyes. If photography is your business, it may be wise to wear contact lenses in order to get rid of the spectacle nuisance.

The viewfinder characteristics of cameras differ. Glasses do not interfere on some as much as others. Keep this in mind when selecting a camera. Check to see if the entire frame is visible when wearing lenses. Individual tolerance varies also. Some photographers do not seem to mind their glasses pressing hard against the camera.

Waist-Level Viewfinders

Cameras focused and framed by looking downward into them at waist level, such as the twin-reflex group, create a different visual problem than do the eye-level variety. The eye must adjust to the camera distance, generally fourteen to twenty inches. This is easy for young eyes which wear the proper distance correction, but for those photographers in their early forties and beyond, the solution then is far from simple. The extra lens power needed to deliver the near focus will interfere with looking at a distance.

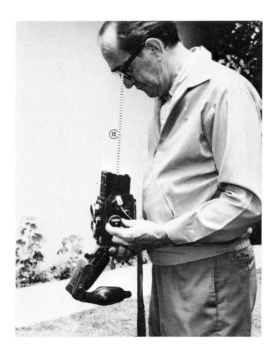

Focusing twin reflex cameras requires sharp near vision at about fourteen to sixteen inches. Some photographers will need a bifocal to do this.

A single vision lens correction can be very nicely used to focus and frame on the ground glass screen. However, such glasses would have to be removed when the photographer is looking directly at the scene or subject. Neither could they be worn when using the sports finder, since it is only an alignment device and requires distance vision.

The waist-level viewfinder requires a bifocal for the greatest convenience even if no distance correction is necessary. Or a half frame could be used if the top edge of the eyeglass frame created no difficulty in looking up or down. The add power must be enough to produce good sharp focus as close as fourteen inches. But to be sure of the distance, each photographer should carefully check the distance from his eye to where he focuses the ground glass screen.

Press and Studio Cameras

Studio and press cameras are focused and framed only nine to fourteen inches from the eyes and straight ahead. The ground glass screen requires critical vision at a closer distance than a person normally works. This must be taken into account when lenses are prescribed. Again, the young eye generally encounters no problem but as near vision blurs with age, the photographer may be in trouble.

The extra power single vision lens required for eye to screen distance will interfere with looking at the subject, as is done in the studio. Yet ordinary bifocals have a drawback too since the near segment is generally too low for viewing the screen without tilting the head back. The answer is a bifocal set very high in the lens; or even better, a lens with only a tiny window at the top for looking at a distance.

Near Vision Problems in Photography

Nearly all cameras require seeing at fourteen to twenty inches to read light meters and set speed and aperture. Since this must often be done quickly or a choice shot is lost, there is little time to switch from one pair of glasses to another. When the bifocal stage arrives, the photographer should wear them and they should be made exactly to his particular needs.

Bifocals fitted for other jobs may not do best for photography. When your vision is examined, describe your photography work in

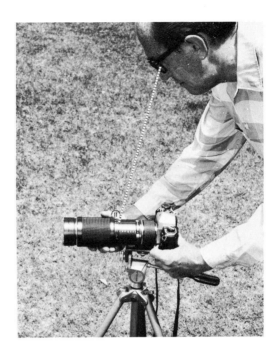

Camera settings may be made as close as ten to twelve inches, and lenses may have to be especially designed for that.

detail. Supply measurements for your working distance—eye to ground glass, to light meter, to film when loading, to scale settings, etc. Even better, take your cameras with you and demonstrate exactly what you do and the kind of viewfinders you use.

Seeing in the Darkroom

The photographer may find that his toughest seeing problems are in the darkroom. The safelight is not enough for good visibility. Make it easiest on your eyes by doing everything you can with normal illumination. You may have trouble in the darkroom even though your eyes work adequately in the light; the reason is that dim images do not provide adequate guidance to the eye's focusing and aiming mechanisms. Glasses may be needed in the darkroom but not elsewhere.

Is your darkroom arranged for easiest seeing in dim light? Critical working areas should be comfortably centered below the eyes, usually sixteen to twenty inches away. Keep papers and materials in well-marked containers where they get illumination from the safelight. Keep everything where it is visually handy.

Enlarging, composing, and framing are generally best done from a twenty- to thirty-inch distance in order to get a good overall view. The bifocal wearer will be in difficulty here since the view is too close to see through the distance portion of lenses and too far away for the bifocal part to be useful (depending upon lens power and available seeing range). Special lenses could be made for this purpose, but moving in closer to get in bifocal range may be easier than changing glasses for this one job. It will, however, restrict the broad view to some degree.

Focusing enlargements is the hardest of all darkroom seeing tasks. To be sure of a sharp image, you should be as close as nine to fourteen inches. Shutting one eye may help momentarily to eliminate the need to converge the two eyes for such a short distance. You can use a magnifier if your glasses do not permit clear vision at that close distance. If you do a lot of enlarging, be sure your glasses permit good seeing at the distance you focus enlargements.

But even with the best glasses a magnifier is almost essential if you want to be absolutely certain of sharp focus. A hand-held, four-inch-diameter magnifier boosts image size about the right amount. Even better are the magnifiers which sit right on the easel and enable you to focus the aerial image of the negative grain. (Inquire at your camera shop about these. One brand is called Magni-Focuser.) And of course, focusing should be done with the aperture stop wide open to get all the light possible.

Special viewing lights should be used to compare picture quality and detail. It is easy to be fooled in the darkroom. For greatest accuracy, your eyes need plenty of light directed specifically on the critical seeing area. But since much ordinary light is not permitted, the photographer must learn to judge sharpness, contrast and detail without it.

A set of good prints should be available for comparison. Take several enlargements with the tonal qualities you prefer and the degree of darkness desired and place them near the developing tray where they can be easily compared with the print being developed. Both are now in the same light, and one is just what you want in normal illumination. The trick of course is to adjust the other under the darkroom safelight to match its appearance.

Retouching calls for the finest of visual discrimination. It is near work of a closer sort than almost any other job or hobby. Eyes must not only be able to focus at a nine- to twelve-inch distance but also to aim together easily and accurately. Glasses may be needed for retouching before they are needed for anything else. Lenses may even have to be made especially for this purpose, or a magnifier used.

Serious photographers have more than one lens for their cameras, and a selection of filters besides. Some have more than one camera. For best vision in photography, several different pairs of glasses could be required for seeing close up or at a distance, in light, or in darkness.

chapter **16**

the sportsman
indoors

Many sportsmen work as hard at their hobbies indoors as out. Repairing equipment, loading cartridges, tying flies, fletching arrows, working on a sailboat or snowmobile—these jobs fill long winter nights and for some can be as enjoyable as the sport itself.

Near vision problems were discussed in Chapters 3 and 6. Much of what was said there applies to the sportsman indoors; these indoor tasks generally require the eyes to be used at close distances, often for long periods of time. Correction of "minor" visual problems may therefore be needed long before these problems cause any difficulty elsewhere.

Only for a brief span in history has man used his eyes for intensive close work during the long hours made possible by artificial light. His ancestors were hunters or farmers, primarily dependent upon their distant vision. Close work is a "recent" invention and the human eye is not yet adapted, if it ever will be, for shopwork and such artificial near seeing tasks.

Good Illumination

Provide good illumination in every critical seeing area.

Lighting for the central working area, whether on bench or machine, should measure at least twenty to thirty foot-candles. That is about the amount supplied by an uncovered 100-watt bulb that is three and a half to four feet away. Depending upon the type of shade or reflector, a work lamp may take as much as 150 watts. At ceiling level, 200 watts or more may be needed to supply that much light.

Hold this book three and a half to four feet from a 100-watt bulb. Note its visibility. Then compare how the print looks in the critical area where you work. It is as easy to read? If not, increase the amount of light until it is.

General room illumination is seldom high enough for critical seeing jobs. It is best to have an adjustable lamp right over the work area as well. Use indirect light if possible to cut shadows and glare. Either fluorescent or incandescent light is satisfactory, so long as you get enough illumination.

Balance

Avoid spotlighting your work. Use balanced lighting.

Two kinds of light are necessary for good sight—specific light on the seeing task and general room illumination. The eye becomes rapidly fatigued when it must work one moment in high brightness, then in the next try to adjust to dimness. A bright spotlight on the work with the rest of the room dark is an arrangement often found in work areas, but it is hard on the eyes. There should be general lighting throughout the workshop and special illumination on the work area.

Glare

Eliminate sources of glare.

Glare is as bad as not enough light. Eyes are attracted to bright areas, and cannot concentrate on the work. Exposed bulbs, all too common in the home workshop, should be shaded. Most modern lamps with bulb covers and reflecting shields minimize glare. Any distracting source of brightness, such as a shiny surface or a window that is too bright, should be eliminated.

Contrast is heightened if you work in your own shadow. Room fixtures are often in the center of the room and create shadows on the workbench. Provide a work lamp, adjustable if possible, to get plenty of light on the critical seeing area and reduce contrasts and glare.

Bright lamps should be shaded. No glare source should be within 45 degrees of the line of sight. Raise the light, change your working area if necessary to get away from direct glare.

The Advantages of Paint

Paint walls, ceilings, benches and floors a light color for better visibility.

Unpainted walls, whether board or cement, generally are too dark or do not reflect enough light for good seeing. Light-colored surfaces diffuse light throughout the room (color is not particularly important as long as it is light). A dull finish is best to prevent annoying reflections and glare.

Your central working area should never be more than three times brighter than the surrounding area. For example, if you work with a shiny metal part on a dark bench or a machine surface, the critical seeing area (the piece itself) will be too much brighter than its background. A paint job helps to brighten surrounding areas and keep down too much contrast. Visibility is much better if working surfaces and surrounding floors and walls are similar in brightness to working materials.

Positioning of Work

Center your work at a height and position for easy focus with each eye.

Eyes work best if they are equidistant from the seeing task. Normal reading position illustrates this nicely—the book is centered on the body, it is well downward from eye level, and is tilted so the page is nearly perpendicular to the line of sight. Tables, jigs, benches,

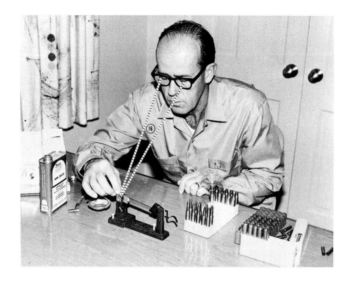

For easy seeing, work should be centered and at a distance of from sixteen to twenty-two inches.

machines should be adjustable to approximate the normal reading situation, even tilted when this is possible.

The average height of power equipment is thirty-six to forty inches. But all home craftsmen are not the same height! Whether you stand or use a stool, have the work area adjustable so that it is necessary to bend over to see at *your* comfortable seeing distance. You can work and see in an abnormal position briefly, but if you stay at it, adjust the work to suit your personal habits.

Eye Protection

Protect your eyes from injury on hazardous operations.

The sportsman who is doing handwork using tools and machines at home runs the risk of eye injury. This is especially true if he is not an expert, for his inexperience prevents him from recognizing the danger. High-speed machines are always a source of danger from a flying object. But hand tools can produce eye injury also—a screw

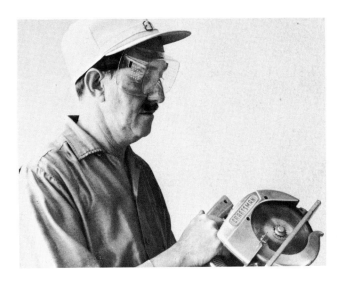

A plastic shield provides good eye protection when using power or hand tools.

driver slips, a hammer sends a nail spinning, or a piece of dust, dirt, wood, or metal flies into the eye.

Simple and inexpensive plastic shields, worn over regular glasses, can provide adequate protection in the average home workshop. Safety goggles made of glass or plastic offer even greater protection. If prescription lenses are necessary, these too can be made in safety form. The person who wears ordinary glasses is in more danger than one who wears none at all.

Organizing Equipment

Arrange tools, supplies, shelves and drawers with visibility in mind.

Difficulties related to near vision problems can be minimized in the arrangement of the workshop. Keep small tools and parts on shelves, or in drawers, within easy arm's reach and never above eye level. Print labels with lettering that is large and clear so you need

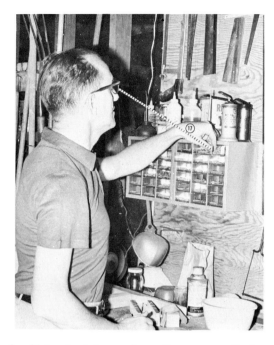

Small items should be kept low, where they can easily be seen through bifocals without head tilt, and they should be in bifocal range.

not get close to read them. Rod repair materials, cartridge loading supplies, and any miniscule objects should be well inside seeing range.

The most difficult seeing area is above the eye level and farther away than twenty-four to thirty-six inches. Put large tools in this area, where they can be seen but do not have to appear perfectly clear. Small ones should be low and close at hand, where they can be spotted through bifocals.

Visual Problems

Be on the lookout for eyes not up to the job.

Your eyes need to focus strongly and accurately for most detail jobs in the home workshop, and they must do this without fatigue. Depending upon your occupation, your hobby may even demand more of your eyes than your regular work. Long hours are often put in on a pet project, after a full day's work. Eyes which get by nicely during an ordinary day may require extra care for a nighttime hobby.

The symptoms of visual problems were discussed in Chapter 3, but any of the following may well indicate deficient eyesight for shop-work: blurred vision of near objects; headache or tiredness clearly associated with use of the eyes; double vision; inability to line things up; errors in cutting, sawing, measuring, and marking, or frequent mistakes of any kind; listlessness and loss of interest.

It is a good idea to rest your eyes occasionally so that fatigue doesn't impair their efficiency. Run through the "tension relievers" described in Chapter 4, but be sure that these relaxing exercises aren't masking some serious eye difficulty which requires professional attention.

Glasses for the Job at Hand

If you wear glasses, be sure they do the job in your workshop.

Measure your actual working distance in inches. The average critical seeing distance is sixteen to eighteen inches, but individual arm length and posture make a difference. Detailed work and fine finishing may be done as close as eleven to twelve inches, while for some jobs good vision is necessary from twenty-two inches to arm's length away. When you have your eyes examined, be prepared to explain exactly what your needs are.

Glasses can be designed to do any specific job, but they may not meet every seeing need once the bifocal stage has been reached. Glasses are a tool, like any other tool, for your hobby. For some eyes, several tools may be needed—possibly trifocals or a specially designed double bifocal with a section at the top of the lens for reading on overhead shelves. Some hobbyists prefer a single vision lens with an intermediate focus for general work and another pair for closer-than-average seeing. Rarely do everyday glasses *fully* meet the needs of the sportsman in his home workshop.

Single vision glasses for close work may be best for some indoor hobby jobs that require very critical seeing—handwork on a gunstock, painting trout lures, polishing stones collected on a hiking trip. Such lenses can be focused for eight to ten inches if necessary.

Another solution to the need for sharp near vision is to use a magnifying device. Stand mounted models are very convenient because they leave the hands free. Loupes, made for use with either one or

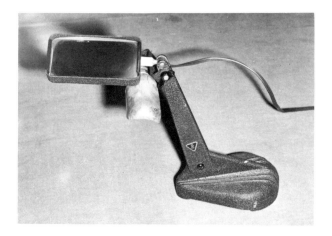

A stand magnifier is handy for doing very fine detail work.

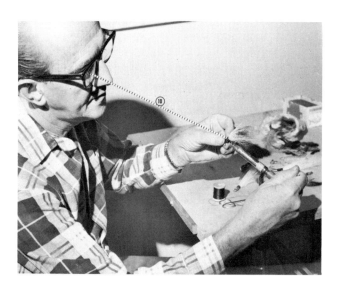

Measure eye-to-work distance for whatever your indoor hobby. This information is critical in getting lenses to do the job.

two, also provide good focus for fine work, especially when natural vision is beginning to slip. Inexpensive magnifiers that fit on a band around the head or attach to spectacles are available.

Remember as pointed out in Chapters 3 and 6, multifocals can be made in almost any power segment combination or position needed. The information needed to produce such a lens should include an exact description of your visual needs and the distances for which each of the lens sections must focus. When you desire the best and go to the trouble of getting the necessary facts, you will achieve more efficient vision for all your sporting needs.

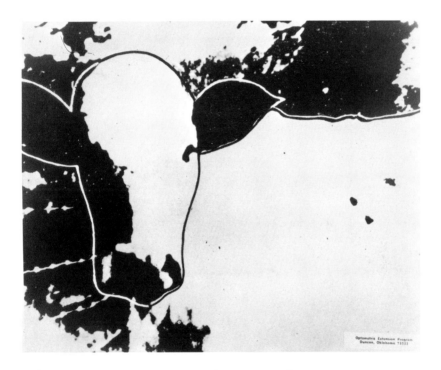

Key to the illustration on page 44. *(Courtesy of the Optometric Extension Program Foundation)*

glossary

Aberration, chromatic. Failure of a lens to bring all light rays to the same point focus because of different refrangibility of light of different colors.

Aberration, spherical. Failure of a lens to bring all light rays to the same point focus because of the lens form which focuses paraxial rays differently than axial rays.

Accommodation. Act of focusing the eye.

Astigmatism. Refractive condition in which there is no point focus because of unequal curvature between the major surface meridians of the optical system.

Aqueous humor. Fluid whch fills the space between cornea and lens of the eye.

Binocular vision. Seeing with both eyes; generally implies seeing a single image.

Coating, lens. Thin deposit of metal, such as magnesium fluoride, applied to a lens surface, which by interference reduces the amount of reflected light. Coating combined with a coloring ingredient also reduces light transmission.

Ciliary muscle. Muscle inside the eye that enables it to change focus.

Concave lens. Diverging lens, also called a minus lens, used to correct nearsightedness.

Cone. Retinal nerve cell which provides sharp visual acuity and color vision.

Convergence. Act of turning the two eyes inward to aim at an object.

Convex lens. Converging lens, also called a plus lens, used to correct far-sightedness.

Cornea. Transparent layer at the front of the eyeball, protective and refractive in function.

Crystalline lens. Lens of the human eye.

Cylindrical lens. Lens used to correct astigmatism; has greater power in one principal meridan than the other.

Dark adaptation. Adjustment of the eye to low level of illumination.

Diopter. Unit of lens power. A one-diopter lens has the power to focus parallel rays of light at a distance of one meter from the lens.

Emmetropia. Refractive condition of the eye; when the eye is completely relaxed, distant objects are in focus on the retina.

Entrance pupil. Pupil or effective aperture through which all rays entering an optical system must pass. An aperture stop on the object side of an optical system.

Error of refraction. See Refractive error.

Exit pupil. Effective aperture through which all light rays must pass when leaving an optical system. An aperture stop on the image side of an optical system.

Extraocular muscles. Muscles which attach to the outside of the eyeball and direct its movements.

Eyebrow relief. Distance between the back edge of a telescopic sight and the eyebrow.

Eye exercises. See Visual training.

Eyepoint. Point behind the back surface of the ocular lens of an optical system, such as binoculars or telescope, where the eye must be placed to get the maximum field of view.

Eye relief. Same as eyebrow relief. Actually the distance from the back lens to the exit pupil of the system.

Farsightedness. See Hyperopia.

Field size, apparent. Angular distance through which the eye must move to look from one edge of a magnified field to the other edge.

Field size, real. Amount of space in degrees which can be seen through an optical system.

Fovea. Small area in center of retina that produces sharpest visual acuity.

Fusion, motor. Process of moving the eyes so that images of a common object are in registry on the two retinas.

Fusion, sensory. Process that blends the two images, one from each eye, into a single mental impression.

Hyperopia. Condition of the eye in which the eye is out of focus for distant objects when focus is at rest; however, vision may be kept clear by accommodation. Also called farsightedness.

Incident light. Rays of light that fall on the eye or an optical system.

Interpupillary distance. Distance between the centers of the pupils of the two eyes.

Iris. Colored diaphragm that moves to control the amount of light entering the eye.

Light efficiency rating. Value sometimes used to designate the brightness of an image produced by an optical system such as binoculars.

Line of sight. Line along which the eye sights in looking at an object, running from the center of the entrance pupil to the object.

Monocular. Seeing with one eye.

Myopia. Eye condition in which the refractive power of the eye is too strong for distant objects, but permits it to see near objects clearly. Also called nearsightedness.

Nearsightedness. *See* Myopia.

Open sight. Iron gunsight in which the back sight is generally a slotted V or W and the front a single post.

Optical center. The most perfect point in an optical system; or, more technically, the only point through which a ray of light can pass and maintain the same direction before and after refraction.

Presbyopia. Decreasing ability of the eye to focus for near objects due to age.

Prism. Wedge-shaped piece of glass which bends light but does not bring it to a focus.

Prismatic effect. Effect of bending light like a prism, also produced by looking through a lens away from its optical center.

Pupil. Aperture in the iris through which light enters the eye.

Refractive error. Expression of the degree to which the eye fails to bring parallel rays of light to exact focus on the retina.

Retina. Inner lining of the eye containing the visual cells which are sensitive to light and many connecting nerve cells.

Rod. Retinal nerve cell specialized for seeing in dim light.

Sclera. Tough, white outer covering of the eyeball.

Spectacle plane. Plane thirteen millimeters in front of the eye where spectacle lenses should be positioned.

Spherical lens. Lens which has spherical faces; each face a smooth polished surface with equal surface curvature in all meridians. Such a lens brings light to a point focus.

Stereopsis. Ability of the brain to coordinate the two slightly disparate images each eye produces; one of the factors contributing to depth perception.

Visual acuity. Measure of the clearness or sharpness of vision.

Visual field. Area of space visible with the human eye.

Visual training. Process of reeducation of visual habits.

Vitreous humor. Jelly-like substance filling the vitreous chamber.